DAIRY CATTLE: WELFARE IN PRACTICE

DAIRY CATTLE: WELFARE IN PRACTICE

Eva Mainau, Déborah Temple, Pol Llonch
and Xavier Manteca

Series Editor: Xavier Manteca

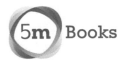
5m Books

First published 2022

Copyright © Eva Mainau, Déborah Temple, Pol Llonch, Xavier Manteca 2022

Published by
5M Books Ltd,
Lings, Great Easton,
Essex CM6 2HH, UK,
Tel: +44 (0)330 1333 580
www.5mbooks.com

A Catalogue record for this book is available from the British Library

ISBN 9781912178353
eISBN 9781789182002
DOI 10.52517/9781789182002

Book layout by KSPM, 8 Wood Road, Codsall, Wolverhampton, WV8 1DB
Printed by Hobbs The Printers Ltd, Totton, Hampshire

Photos and illustrations by the authors unless otherwise indicated

Contents

Contributors

Pol Llonch – Department of Animal and Food Science, School of Veterinary Science, Universitat Autònoma de Barcelona, 08193 Bellaterra (Barcelona), Spain

Eva Mainau – AWEC Advisors SL, Ed. Eureka, Parc de Recerca UAB, 08193 Bellaterra (Barcelona), Spain

Xavier Manteca – Department of Animal and Food Science, School of Veterinary Science, Universitat Autònoma de Barcelona, 08193 Bellaterra (Barcelona), Spain

Déborah Temple – AWEC Advisors SL, Ed. Eureka, Parc de Recerca UAB, 08193 Bellaterra (Barcelona), Spain

Foreword

Animal welfare is largely perceived as a 'public good' by society, and it is considered a necessary element of sustainable animal production. It is also associated with other aspects, such as animal health, productivity, and efficiency from a cost-of-production perspective. Therefore, animal welfare is an essential tool to gain and maintain markets, and any husbandry that benefits sustainability should maximize animal welfare and avoid its potential impairment. To help ensure public confidence, the on-site assessment of welfare as well as the implementation of 'best practice' standards should be based on a solid scientific background.

Dairy Cattle: Animal Welfare in Practice, structured in 10 chapters, translates the scientific knowledge of the welfare of dairy cattle into practice. The book includes definitions of animal welfare and key scientific approaches to welfare issues related to feeding, housing, health, and behaviour. These chapters provide a scientifically based outline for how to evaluate the welfare of dairy cattle at a farm level. They pay special attention to the animal-based measures, although other environmentally based and management-based parameters are also described. The later chapters focus on the most pressing welfare challenges in dairy cattle, such as milking, drying-off, calving, and pre-weaning. The emphasis is not just on discussing problems, but on identifying strategies for improving welfare. These issues are elaborated by well-known experts in their field. This unique approach has added value compared with other books because of the practical approach and experience in field work.

The onus of maintaining good animal welfare is on the farmers, veterinarians, and assessors who are required to put in place monitoring procedures, including animal-based indicators, to evaluate animal welfare, and housing and management strategies to ensure the welfare of dairy cattle. This will be a reference book of valuable practical information that veterinarians, practitioners, farmers, and veterinary and animal science students can use to identify welfare problems and to improve animal welfare on dairy farms. The book will not only help improve dairy cattle welfare but also encourage discussion about future priorities and solutions.

Dr Antonio Velarde Calvo

European Veterinary Specialist in Animal Welfare Science, Ethics and Law by the ECAWBM (European College of Animal Welfare and Behaviour Medicine)

Head of the Animal Welfare programme at IRTA (Institute of Agrifood Research and Technology)

CHAPTER 1

What is animal welfare?

1.1 Characteristics of animal welfare

The concept of animal welfare includes three main elements: the animal's **normal biological functioning** (which, among other things, means ensuring that the animal is healthy and well nourished), its **emotional state** (including the absence of negative emotions such as pain and chronic fear and the presence of positive emotions), and its **ability to express certain behaviours** (Figure 1.1). These three principles are often complementary. This notwithstanding, not all behaviours are equally important in terms of animal welfare. From a practical standpoint, the clearest indication that a given behaviour is important is whether the animal shows a stress response or exhibits abnormal behaviour when prevented from performing it. A calf's sucking behaviour is an example of such an important behaviour.

Animal welfare can be assessed on the basis of each of the three main elements. The first approach assesses an animal's welfare based on the

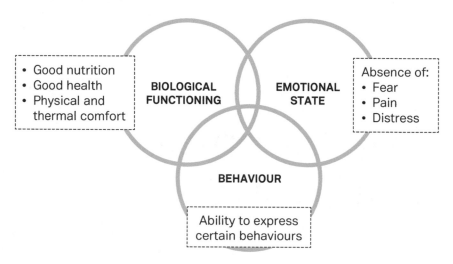

Figure 1.1 Main elements that determine animal welfare (adapted from Fraser et al., 1997).

presence of an adequate biological function. To cope with a challenge, the animal will activate various body-repair systems, immunological defences, physiological stress responses, and several behavioural responses. The biological cost of these responses can ultimately affect the growth, health, and reproduction of the animal.

The second approach links welfare to the absence of negative emotions and the presence of positive ones. Concerns for animal welfare are generally based on the assumption that animals can subjectively experience emotional states and, hence, can suffer or experience pleasure. European legislation (the Treaty of Amsterdam) refers to animals as 'sentient beings' (Council of the European Union, 1997). The suffering of individual animals is often a concern of the general public, and nowadays most scientists accept that animal suffering, and the degree of animal consciousness that this implies, are essential aspects of animal welfare.

Finally, some definitions of welfare are based on the ability of the animals to engage in normal patterns of behaviour. 'Normal behaviour' is usually associated with the behaviour shown by most members of a species under natural conditions. Defining what should be considered normal or not (or, conversely, prejudicial or not) for the animal is not straightforward, especially when dealing with animals housed in a variety of conditions. However, it is accepted that welfare is impaired when the inability of an animal to show a particular behaviour results in pain or suffering. Such behaviours are usually known as **behavioural needs**.

These apparently divergent definitions of welfare are, in fact, **three complementary issues**. Each of these approaches has its own merits but none of them captures on its own the different aspects of animal welfare. It has been suggested, therefore, that the assessment of animal welfare should include all three approaches, and all three principles are included in multiple 'official' definitions of animal welfare.

World Organisation for Animal Health (OIE) Terrestrial Animal Health Code (2021)

Animal welfare means the physical and mental state of an animal in relation to the conditions in which it lives and dies. An animal experiences good welfare if the animal is healthy, comfortable, well nourished, safe, does not suffering from unpleasant states, such as pain, fear and distress, and is able to express behaviours that are important for its physical and mental state.

Welfare can vary over a wide range, from very good to very poor. In between these extremes, the animal may cope with a given situation, but with a cost of adaptation. Welfare depends on whether the animal is able to cope, and on how much it has to do to cope, with challenges in its environment. As feelings are part of the coping mechanisms used by animals, feelings are an important part of welfare.

'The term welfare refers to the state of an individual in relation to its environment, and this can be measured' (Donald Broom, animal welfare scientist).

The animal reaches a state of good welfare when it is kept in an environment that allows it to satisfy its motivations and enables it to experience positive emotional states. When the situation moves away from this ideal state, the animal will use a wide range of physiological mechanisms and behaviours to cope with its environment. The ability to cope successfully or not will depend on the individual animal itself and on how much it must cope with. The inability to cope with an adverse situation may lead to the appearance of injury or disease, and consequently to pain and suffering.

1.2 The Five Freedoms

In accordance with the Five Freedoms principle, an animal's welfare is ensured when the following five conditions are met (FAWC, 1979, 1993):

- The animal is free from hunger, thirst, and malnutrition, because it has ready access to drinking water and a suitable diet.
- The animal is free from physical and thermal discomfort, because it has access to shelter from the elements and a comfortable resting area.
- The animal is free from pain, injury, and disease, thanks to suitable prevention and/or rapid diagnosis and treatment.
- The animal is able to express most of its normal behavioural patterns, because it has sufficient space, proper facilities, and the company of other animals of its kind.
- The animal does not experience fear or distress, because the conditions needed to prevent mental suffering have been ensured.

The Five Freedoms principle offers a very useful and practical approach to the study of animal welfare, and especially to its assessment on livestock farms and during the transport and slaughter of farm animals. It provides a checklist by which to assess the strengths and weaknesses of husbandry systems. It has, moreover, served as the basis for many animal-protection laws in the European Union and other parts of the world. However, despite its clear usefulness, it has two shortcomings. First, it is sometimes too generic. Second, there is a degree of overlap between some of the Five Freedoms. To remedy these problems, slightly different approaches based on the same concepts have been proposed. Of particular note is the Welfare Quality® project's proposal for assessing animal welfare (www.welfarequality.net). The Welfare Quality® project was a 5-year European Union research project launched in May 2004 and involving more than 40 scientific institutions from 15 different countries. One of its objectives was to develop European standards for animal welfare assessment. Unlike other protocols, which mainly use environment-based parameters, the protocols of the Welfare Quality® project are primarily founded on animal-based measures.

1.3 Beyond the Five Freedoms

The Five Domains Model goes beyond the Five Freedoms by giving more importance to positive emotions and their impact on the overall welfare state of the animal. This model incorporates four main domains related to the biological and physical functioning of the animal (nutrition, environment, health, and behaviour) and a fifth domain related to affective/mental experiences. Each one of these domains can be negatively or positively affected. The model takes a predominantly physiological perspective, and is structured to initially assess particular physical or functional disruptions and imbalances, as well as restrictions on the expression of important behaviours. It then identifies the likely specific negative effects resulting from each disruption, imbalance, or behavioural restriction. The overall affective outcome in the 'mental' domain represents the overall welfare status of the animal (Table 1.1).

To improve the welfare of animals, it is necessary, overall, to minimize their negative experiences and, at the same time, to provide the animals with opportunities to have positive experiences. Barren, isolated conditions, and unpredictable or threatening situations should be avoided and

Table 1.1 The Five Domains Model (adapted from Mellor, 2016).

Nutrition		Environment		Health		Behaviour	
–	+	–	+	–	+	–	+
Restricted water and food	Good quality and quantity of food and water	Discomfort	Physical environment comfortable	Diseases and injuries	Healthy	Restrictions of important behaviours	Expression of important behaviours

Mental affective state	
–	+
Thirst and hunger Cold or overheating Pain and sickness Frustration Boredom, loneliness Anxiety, fear, panic, exhaustion	Drinking and taste pleasures, satiety Physical comfort Health and fitness Rewarding experiences Goal-directed motivations Calm and in control Positive social behaviour Maternal behaviour Sexual behaviour Play

Note: –, negative factors; +, positive factors.

replaced by stimulus-rich and safe environments that provide opportunities for the animals to engage in behaviours they find rewarding.

Attitudes and good management are key features to improve animal welfare

The quality of stockpersons is fundamental to ensure proper welfare of the animals they manage. Under intensive conditions, stockpeople have complete control over food and water availability and quality, as well as other resources such as space, comfortable resting places, social groupings, and environmental complexity. Animal-care personnel should anticipate problems, identify when a problem has occurred, and apply solutions as soon as possible. The decisions and behaviours of the persons working with animals have the potential to both compromise and enhance animal welfare. Clearly, the stockperson's personality, attitudes, knowledge, skills, training, and experience with the animals are key elements to positively improve animal welfare. Broader issues such as job motivation and satisfaction, working conditions, and external technical support are important components that will facilitate proper management.

Bibliography

Broom, D.M. (1991) Animal welfare. Concepts and measurements. *Journal of Animal Science* 69, 4167–4175.

Broom, D.M. and Johnson, K.G. (1993) *Stress and Animal Welfare,* 2nd edn. Chapman and Hall, London, UK.

Council of the European Union (1997) Treaty of Amsterdam amending the Treaty on European Union, the Treaties establishing the European Communities and certain related acts. OJ C 340/1. Available at: https://eur-lex.europa.eu/legal-content/EN/TXT/?uri = CELEX:11997D/TXT (accessed 18 October 2021).

FAWC (1979) Farm Animal Welfare Council Press Statement, 5 December 1979. Available at: https://webarchive.nationalarchives.gov.uk/ukgwa/20121007104210/http:/www.fawc.org.uk/pdf/fivefreedoms1979.pdf (accessed 22 November 2021).

FAWC (1993) Second Report on Priorities for Research and Development in Farm Animal Welfare. Surbiton, UK: Farm Animal Welfare Council.

Fraser, D., Weary, D.M., Pajor, E.A. and Milligan, B.N. (1997) A scientific conception of animal welfare that reflects ethical concerns. *Animal Welfare* 6, 187–205.

Hughes, B.O. and Duncan, I.J.H. (1988) The notion of ethological 'need', models of motivation and animal welfare. *Animal Behaviour* 36, 1696–1707.

Mellor, D.J. (2016) Updating animal welfare thinking: moving beyond the 'Five Freedoms' towards 'A life worth living'. *Animals*, 6, 21–40.

Mendl, M. (2001) Animal husbandry: assessing the welfare state. *Nature* 410, 31–32.

OIE (2021) Introduction to the recommendations for animal welfare. In: Terrestrial Animal Health Code 2021. OIE, Paris, France. Available at: https://www.oie.int/en/what-we-do/standards/codes-and-manuals/terrestrial-code-online-access/ (accessed 22 November 2021).

Spinka, M. (2006) How important is natural behaviour in animal farming systems? *Applied Animal Behaviour Science* 100, 117–128.

CHAPTER 2

How can animal welfare be assessed?

Welfare is multidimensional and it cannot be measured directly and by a single measure. Rather, animal welfare science is multidisciplinary and makes use of a great variety of parameters. These parameters can be categorized into two main types: environment-based and animal-based measures.

2.1 Environment-based and animal-based measures

It is possible to assess the welfare of animals by looking at their environment. Resource- and management-based measures (**inputs**) can indicate whether the environment is acceptable for the animals. Resource-based measures include, for example, the dimensions of the feeding area, the number of drinking places, the dimensions of the resting area (e.g.

cubicle), and the quality of the resting area. The feeding management of calves (the quantity and type of milk, method of milk provision, and number of meals per day) is an example of a management-based measure. These indirect measures of welfare are based on assumptions concerning the relationships between aspects of the environment and the actual welfare state of the animals. Environment-based factors are fundamental for the provision of advice concerning the prevention of a welfare problem and for the detection of a risk of deficient welfare. Information on the risk of welfare problems is particularly important to detect problems that occur rarely.

Instead of measuring the provision of good husbandry, welfare can be measured by observing the animal directly. Animal-based measures (**outcomes**) indicate the effect of the indirect, environment-based measures and their interactions with the animal. Since welfare is a condition of the animal, animal-based measures are likely to provide the most direct information on its welfare state. Therefore, they are generally considered to be more valid measures of welfare than environment-based measures, and they should be applicable across production systems. Animal-based measures involve both animal observations and the use of farm records of the animals and fall into five main categories: performance, health, physiology, behaviour, and post-mortem measurements (Figure 2.1).

'Animal-based measures are considered more valid than environment-based measures for the assessment of animal welfare.'

Environment- and animal-based measures present both advantages and disadvantages. Consequently, the combination of both types of parameters gives the most valid and complete assessment of animal welfare and enables one not only to assess the current welfare state of the animals but also to evaluate potential risks to their welfare.

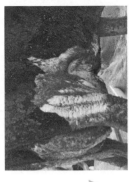

Facilities (e.g. cubicle size)

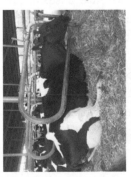

Management
(e.g. bed maintenance)

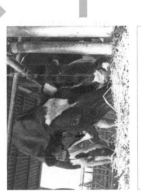

**Characteristics of
the cow** (genetics,
health, production,
temperament, etc.)

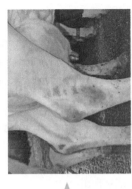

Cleanliness of the cow

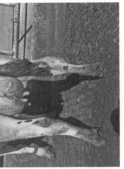

Lesions of the hock

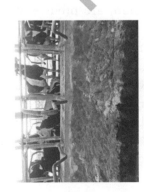

Hock swelling

Figure 2.1 Example of environment-based and animal-based measures related to
cow comfort around resting. Cubicle size and maintenance of the bed (inputs) are
risk factors that contribute to the cleanliness of the cows, and to the presence of
hair patches, lesions and swellings of the hock (outcomes).

2.1.1 The Welfare Quality® protocols

The Welfare Quality® (WQ) protocols (www.welfarequality.net) can be considered as a reference method for the overall assessment of animal welfare. The WQ protocol for dairy cattle provides a tool to assess animal welfare in a standardized way.

According to WQ, animal welfare assessments must take the following four questions into account.

- Are the animals properly fed?
- Are the animals properly housed?
- Are the animals healthy?
- Does the behaviour of the animals reflect optimal emotional states?

The last of these questions may be the most innovative and controversial aspect. In brief, it refers to the fact that animals should not experience fear, pain, frustration, or any other negative emotional state, at least chronically or in a very intense way.

The four questions give rise to a set of 12 criteria on which any welfare assessment system should be based. For each of these criteria, several measures were selected. Most of these measures are based on the direct observation of the animal (i.e. they are animal-based measures) (Table 2.1).

Parallel to the WQ, there are other systems of welfare assessment based on measurements of animals. For example, the Bristol Welfare Assurance Programme (BWAP) contributed to the development of Advancing Animal Welfare Assurance (Assurewel; www.assurewel.org/dairycows.html). CowSignals® (www.cowsignals.com) has been developed by a team of dairy experts in The Netherlands and is an illustrated guide for farmers and veterinarians on how to interpret the behaviour, posture, and physical characteristics of cows.

Table 2.1 Summary of the principles, criteria, and measures of the Welfare Quality® protocol for dairy cows.

Principles	Criteria	Measures
Good feeding	Absence of prolonged hunger	Body condition score
	Absence of prolonged thirst	Water supply
Good housing	Comfort around resting	Behaviours around resting, cleanliness of the body
	Thermal comfort	As yet, no measure has been developed (panting is under revision)
	Ease of movement	Presence of tethering Access to outdoor loafing area
Good health	Absence of injuries	Lameness, integument alterations
	Absence of disease	Respiratory, enteric, reproductive disorders Mortality, dystocia, downer cows
	Absence of pain induced by management procedures	Dehorning (procedure and protocol for anaesthesia and analgesia) Tail docking (performed or not)
Appropriate behaviour	Expression of social behaviours	Agonistic behaviours
	Expression of other behaviours	Access to pasture
	Good human–animal relationship	Avoidance distance at feeding place
	Positive emotional state	Qualitative Behaviour Assessment

2.2 Performance measures

The accumulation of all attempts to cope with several challenging situations will ultimately affect the animal, and thus its performance. It is worth noting that good performance is not a guarantee of optimized welfare. An examination of performance records can give a first general approximation of the welfare state of the animals on a farm. Performance parameters give an overview of the problems that a herd may experience over time. For example, a high culling rate (uncontrolled culling) can indicate that cows are suffering from several undesirable diseases or injuries that ultimately hasten their death. Similarly, the mortality rate of dairy calves reflects the number of animals becoming so sick that they die before slaughter. If two animal husbandry systems are compared and the mortality rate is significantly higher in the first than in the second system, then we can say that animal welfare is poorer in the first system. Poor reproductive performance in cows can be linked to stress situations as well as many other factors that are not directly related to welfare (e.g. oestrus detection, timing of insemination, storage of semen). The main limitation of performance measures is their lack of specificity, which makes them difficult to interpret. However, Table 2.2 proposes a list of performance parameters to take into consideration when assessing the welfare of dairy cows.

Table 2.2 Performance parameters and treatment records that can be used by farmers and veterinarians as key indicators of welfare in dairy cows.

Average daily milk production per cow (l/day/cow)
Average milk protein content (%)
Average milk fat content (%)
Average number of lactations per cow
Average lactation length (days)
Average calving-to-conception interval (days)
Average length of dry period (days)

Percentage of herd pregnant by 150 days in milk (%)

Average number of inseminations per pregnancy

Number of eligible cows not inseminated at first-service insemination deadline

Proportion of pregnant cows (%)

Conception rate by service and according to lactation number

Average age of cows at first delivery

Abortions and stillbirths (%)

Dystocia (%)

Caesarean section rate (%)

Average age of cows

Proportion of culled cows (%)

Proportion of voluntarily culled cows (%)

Proportion of involuntarily culled cows (%)

Proportion of 'downer' cows (euthanized on farm) (%)

2.3 Health measures

Health is a very important part of animal welfare and must be properly considered when assessing welfare. In fact, health problems are among the most severe welfare problems for farm animals. Diseases and injuries produce pain and discomfort and can also interfere with the expression of normal patterns of behaviours such as drinking, feeding, and resting. Additionally, the presence of some diseases provides relevant information on the overall quality of the environment in which the animal lives, and this is particularly true for the so-called multifactorial diseases. Some diseases are caused by a well-defined primary pathological agent that plays the most important role, by far, in the incidence and severity of the disease. Bovine viral diarrhoea–mucosal disease

(BVD-MD) and infectious bovine rhinotracheitis (IBR) are examples of such diseases. In contrast, other types of diseases (i.e. multifactorial diseases) are highly dependent on the environment. The impact of these diseases largely depends on a combination of several management, housing, and hygienic conditions on the farm. For such multifactorial diseases, roughly speaking, the presence of a causative agent is a necessary but not sufficient cause for disease. The animal's stress response and the associated immunosuppression resulting from difficulties in coping with the environment have been shown to increase the incidence of these diseases. Examples of common multifactorial diseases in dairy cattle are mastitis, bovine respiratory disease complex, diarrhoea in calves and lameness. As multifactorial diseases and injuries are considered to reflect the overall quality of the environment of the animals, they should be carefully considered within a health assessment system.

2.4 Physiological measures

When an animal tries to cope or fails to cope with several challenges, this induces changes in its physiological parameters (Table 2.3).

Activation of the sympathetic nervous system following a stressful stimulus in an animal may be measured directly by the concentrations of certain hormones (e.g. the catecholamines adrenaline (epinephrine) and noradrenaline (norepinephrine)) or indirectly by the respiratory rhythm, heart rate and its variability, the diameter of the pupil, blood pressure, body temperature, or the plasma concentration of energy metabolites (e.g. lactate, glucose, fatty acids). The sympathetic system is very sensitive to stimuli that are perceived as a threat, and response times are generally short. This system is activated by painful stimuli and also by other stressors such as handling or changes in the environment.

Hypothalamic–pituitary–adrenal (HPA) axis activity, which regulates the release of the glucocorticoid hormone cortisol, has been widely used as an indicator of stress. The release of glucocorticoids can be

Table 2.3 Main biomarkers used to quantify stress and welfare in dairy cattle.

Endocrine measures	
Cortisol	Hypothalamic–pituitary–adrenal
Corticotropin-releasing hormone (CRH)	Hypothalamic–pituitary–adrenal
Adrenocorticotropic hormone (ACTH)	Hypothalamic–pituitary–adrenal
Adrenaline and noradrenaline	Sympathetic adrenal medullary
Vasopressin	Antidiuretic hormone
β-endorphins	Opioid neuropeptide
Biochemical markers	
Non-esterified fatty acids	
β-hydroxybutyrate	
Acute phase proteins	
Urea	
Glucose	
Creatine kinase	
Lactate	
Lactate dehydrogenase	

monitored non-invasively via the measurement of metabolites excreted in urine and faeces, and in saliva and hair. Chronic fear linked to a poor human–animal relationship, painful husbandry practices such as dehorning, or social stress due to competition at the feeding place are examples of challenges that have been associated with an increase in HPA activity. However, how chronic stress affects the activity of the HPA axis still remains unclear. There are still some disagreements among the scientific community on how housing methods affect the levels of glucocorticoids.

The quantification of **acute phase proteins (APPs)** has been used to monitor inflammatory processes in farm animals. It has recently been recognized that animal APP concentrations are useful not only for monitoring inflammatory processes but also for assessing various non-inflammatory conditions, such as pregnancy, parturition, metabolic diseases, and stress. The level of APPs in the plasma has been demonstrated to be useful in the assessment of animal welfare. APP concentrations have been used, for example, to identify the presence of diseases, lesions, and stress linked to long periods of transport or to rearing conditions.

Physiological indicators can be particularly useful in prey species, such as cattle, that are considered stoic and are unlikely to show pronounced behavioural responses until injuries or diseases are severe. Nevertheless, before considering physiological parameters in a welfare assessment, it is important to be aware of some of their limitations. First, physiological changes are difficult to interpret and are not always associated with poor welfare. Similar changes in physiological responses can occur in situations of opposite affective states. Cortisol levels, for example, may rise both in fear-inducing situations and in response to sexual activity. Second, there is usually an important variability between individuals and some parameters may exhibit a circadian pattern. Physiological parameters are also limited in terms of their feasibility. Finally, sample collection for measurement of these parameters usually requires methods that are more or less invasive, as well as special equipment. It must also be considered that the stress caused to the animals during handling for sample collection may reduce the validity of the data.

2.5 Behavioural measures

Behaviour can be a sensitive indicator of the animal's perception of its environment. Variations in behavioural patterns often represent the first level of response of an animal to an averse or stressful environment. When an animal is confronted by environmental challenges, it may react in one or more of the following ways, all of which are indicators of impaired welfare.

- **Changes in the frequency or timing of normal behaviours**. For example, changes in activity levels or a decrease in social behaviours and time spent feeding may indicate an underlying pathology.
- **Problem-specific behavioural changes**. For example, animals adopt pain-specific behaviours to avoid stimulating a painful body area.
- **Expression of abnormal behaviours**, such as redirected behaviours or stereotypes.

Behaviours associated with physical suffering clearly indicate poor welfare. Behaviour is commonly used in the clinical assessment of health and is also considered as the most commonly used parameter to assess pain. The detection of behavioural changes is particularly important both in the diagnosis of a subclinical problem and thereafter in the prevention and control of disease. Behavioural indicators of pain represent a practical way to assess welfare. When a cow is suffering, it generally stands with the neckline, head, and ears in a low position, the back arched, and the tail held close against the hindquarters.

> *'Behavioural measures are considered the most valid and specific parameters when studying pain in animals.'*

Vocalizations can also be used to identify pain. It has been shown that changes in their frequency and intensity can indicate a painful situation. Reluctance to move and a lack of normal social behaviour can be signs of pain related to diseases or injuries. For example, dairy cows reduce their locomotor activity by 70–90% when suffering from visceral pain. Accelerometers, such as pedometers, can be very useful to detect animals with an underlying pathology. Several scales to identify and qualitatively measure pain have been developed and can be practical to use under commercial conditions. The Sprecher lameness-scoring system (Sprecher et al., 1997) and the WQ scoring system for integument alterations are two examples of practical scales. Recently, a Cow Pain

Scale (Gleerup et al., 2015; Gleerup, 2017) that includes several selected behavioural variables, such as attention towards the surroundings, head position, ear position, facial expressions, response to approach, and back position, has been proposed as a means to identify cows that are in pain.

In addition to pain-related behaviours, other changes in the duration and frequency of normal behaviours are recognized as indicators of mental suffering (e.g. frustration). Possible signs of stress include startle or defence responses, avoidance, suppression of feeding and sexual behaviour, excessive aggression, stereotypic behaviour, lack of responsiveness or apathy, decreased complexity of behaviour, and the time required to restart normal activity after experiencing a stressor.

Preventing an animal from carrying out a certain type of behaviour in a given situation might cause signs of suffering. Redirected sucking behaviour in dairy calves linked to a lack of normal sucking behaviour is clearly an abnormal behaviour that may lead to pain. It should be accepted, then, that sucking behaviour in calves is a very important behaviour (i.e. a 'behavioural need') and that assessment of the frequency of redirected sucking behaviour in calves and the quality of feeding management of calves can be used as indicators of welfare. The inability to display certain important behaviours can also manifest itself in the appearance of stereotypic behaviours. An animal performing a stereotypic behaviour repeats a relatively invariant sequence of actions, which has no obvious function. Tongue-rolling is an example of a stereotypic behaviour shown by cattle.

Precision livestock farming

Precision livestock farming (PLF) technology has great potential to monitor behavioural parameters or indicators of animal welfare. Technological and biotechnological innovations in automated health diagnostics are being developed and represent a huge step forward in health monitoring. Biosensors have been developed to detect markers for ovulation, pregnancy, milk lactose concentration, mastitis, and metabolic changes. Wireless telemetry has been applied to develop boluses for monitoring the rumen pH and body temperature to detect metabolic disorders. Lameness can be detected by walking cows through load cells that measure weight distribution, and also by various types of video image analysis and speed measurement. The prediction and detection of calving time is an area of active research mostly focused on behavioural changes. Technological developments are following two different lines: one is to load more sensors onto the animal, particularly on to collars; the other approach, which is inherently cheaper, particularly for large herds, is to have a single monitoring station close to or at the milking system, through which all cows must pass.

Bibliography

Berckmans, D. (2014) Precision livestock farming technologies for welfare management in intensive livestock systems. *OIE Scientific and Technical Review* 33, 189–196.

Blokhuis, H.J., Jones, R.B., Geers, R., Miele, M. and Veissier, I. (2003) Measuring and monitoring animal welfare: transparency in the food product quality chain. *Animal Welfare* 12, 445–455.

Boissy, A., Manteuffel, G., Jensen, M.B., Moe, R.O., Spruijt, B., Keeling, L.J., Winckler, C., Forkman, B., Dimitrov, I., Langbein, J., Bakken, M., Veissier, I. and Aubert, A. (2007) Assessment of positive emotions in animals to improve their welfare. *Physiology and Behavior* 92, 375–397.

Botreau, R., Veissier, I., Butterworth, A., Bracke, M.B.M. and Keeling, L.J. (2007) Definition of criteria for overall assessment of animal welfare. *Animal Welfare* 16, 225–228.

Capdeville, J. and Veissier, I. (2001) A method of assessing welfare in loose housed dairy cows at farm level, focusing on animal observations. *Acta Agriculturae Scandinavica, Section A – Animal Science* 51, 62–68.

Cray, C., Zaias, J. and Altman, N.H. (2009) Acute phase response in animals: a review. *Comparative Medicine* 59, 517–526.

de Rosa, G., Tripaldi, C., Napolitano, F., Grasso, F., Bisegna, V. and Bordi, V. (2003) Repeatability of some animal related variables in dairy cows and buffaloes. *Animal Welfare* 12, 625–629.

Eckersall, P.D., Young, F.J., Nolan, A.M., Knight, C.H., McComb, C., Waterston, M.M., Hogarth, C.J., Scott, E.M. and Fitzpatrick, J.L. (2006) Acute phase proteins in bovine milk in an experimental model of *Staphylococcus aureus* subclinical mastitis. *Journal of Dairy Science* 89, 1488–1501.

Endres, M.I., Lobeck-Luchterhand, K.M., Espejo, L.A. and Tucker, C.B. (2014) Evaluation of the sample needed to accurately estimate outcome-based measurements of dairy welfare on farm. *Journal of Dairy Science* 97, 3523–3530.

Engel, B.G., Bruin, G., Andre, G. and Buist, W. (2003) Assessment of observer performance in a subjective scoring system: visual classification of the gait of cows. *Journal of Agricultural Science* 140, 317–333.

Gleerup, K.B. (2017) Identifying pain behaviors in dairy cattle. In: *Proceedings of the Western Canadian Dairy Seminar: Advances in Dairy Technology, Session VI: Cow Management and Welfare* 29, 231–239.

Gleerup, K.B., Andersen, P.H., Munksgaard, L. and Forkman, B. (2015) Pain evaluation in dairy cattle. *Applied Animal Behaviour Science* 171, 25–32.

Johnsen, P.F., Johannesson, T. and Sandøe, P. (2001) Assessment of farm animal welfare at herd level: many goals, many methods. *Acta Agriculturae Scandinavica, Section A – Animal Science* 51, 26–33.

Knierim, U. and Winckler, C. (2009) On-farm welfare assessment in cattle: validity, reliability and feasibility issues and future perspectives with special regard to the Welfare Quality® approach. *Animal Welfare* 18, 451–458.

Main, D.C.J., Kent, J.P., Wemelsfelder, F., Ofner, E. and Tuyttens, F.A.M. (2003) Applications for methods of on-farm welfare assessment. *Animal Welfare* 12, 523–528.

Mottram, T. (2016) Animal board invited review: Precision livestock farming for dairy cows with a focus on oestrus detection. *Animal* 10, 1575–1584.

Rushen, J. (1991) Problems associated with the interpretation of physiological data in the assessment of animal-welfare. *Applied Animal Behaviour Science* 28, 381–386.

Rushen, J. (2003) Changing concepts of farm animal welfare: bridging the gap between applied and basic research. *Applied Animal Behaviour Science* 81, 199–214.

Rushen, J. and de Passillé, A.M. (1992) The scientific assessment of the impact of housing on animal welfare: a critical review. *Canadian Journal of Animal Science* 72, 721–743.

Sprecher, D.J., Hostetler, D.E. and Kaneene, J.B. (1997) A lameness scoring system that uses posture and gait to predict dairy cattle reproductive performance. *Theriogenology* 47, 1179–1187.

Stygar, A.H., Gómez, Y., Berteselli, G.V., Dalla Costa, E., Canali, E., Niemi, J.K., Llonch, P. and Pastell, M. (2021). A systematic review on commercially available and validated sensor technologies for welfare assessment of dairy cattle. *Frontiers in Veterinary Science* 8, 634338.

Webster, A.J.F. (2005) The assessment and implementation of animal welfare: theory into practice. *OIE Scientific and Technical Review* 24, 723–734.

Webster, A.J.F., Main, D.C.J. and Whay, H.R. (2004) Welfare assessment: indices from clinical observation. *Animal Welfare* 13, 93–98.

CHAPTER 3

Welfare issues related to feeding

Dairy cows in intensive farming systems have shown substantially improved milk yields in recent years. This has resulted from the diets fed to cows having an **increased nutrient density**, which has been primarily achieved by feeding more concentrates and less forages, increasing the **risk of ruminal acidosis**. In addition, dairy cows in confined systems are exposed to **competition for resources**, which may result in some cows being **undernourished**. The welfare problems associated with feeding practices, such as acidosis and undernutrition, can also have notable consequences for productivity.

3.1 Factors regulating feeding behaviour

In ruminants, feeding is a predominant behaviour, and they spend a large proportion of the day feeding (around 8 h a day). In cattle, feeding occurs mostly around dawn and dusk. This time dedicated to feeding is usually associated with the intake of large quantities of feed. Ruminants need to eat a large amount of feed, as the efficiency of converting fibrous feed to nutrients is low. For example, a high-producing dairy cow can eat more than 25 kg of dry matter in a day. In the rumen, the feed is fermented by ruminal microbiota, which are able to digest fibre and make nutrients digestible. In ruminants, feeding is followed by the process of rumination, in which the rumen content is regurgitated to be chewed again. The word 'ruminant' comes from the Latin *ruminare*, meaning 'to chew over again'. This repeated chewing decreases the size of feed particles and makes them more accessible to the ruminal microbiota.

Animals, including ruminants, regulate feeding through the antagonistic motivations of **appetite** and **satiety**. Appetite refers to the subjective desire to eat, which is usually driven by hunger. The most obvious conditions that provoke hunger, and therefore stimulate eating, are energy deficit and weight loss induced by feed deprivation. Hunger should thus be considered as a necessary state to motivate eating, which, per se, is not detrimental to animal welfare. However, if hunger persists, it is converted into a negative subjective indicator of welfare as a result of chronic undernourishment.

Social behaviour has a modulatory effect on feeding. One example is social facilitation, in which an animal's desire to eat is stimulated by the presence of other animals eating. According to this process, when a cow eats, it may stimulate other cows to eat as well, whether they are hungry or not. By contrast, hierarchy and competition between cows mediates feeding, as it determines the access of cows to feed. Hierarchy is present in all herds and leads to a social structure with dominant cows (those with a higher social rank, which access resources first) and subordinate cows (those lower in the social ranking, which access resources last). In situations of limited access to feed, dominant cows may restrict the access of subordinate cows to the feeding place, leading to part of the herd being undernourished.

'Ruminal acidosis and undernutrition are the main welfare problems related to feeding in dairy cattle, and can result in an important loss of productivity.'

3.2 Health and welfare problems derived from feeding

3.2.1 Chronic hunger and state of negative energy balance

In dairy cattle, **chronic hunger** (which leads to an undernourished state) is rare, as cows are usually provided with *ad libitum* feed throughout their production lifetime. On rare occasions, chronic hunger can arise in barns where either the feed is restricted or the dominant–subordinate relationships prevent some cows from accessing the feed in a normal manner. Chronic hunger is a negative emotional status that impairs the welfare of cows. In other situations (e.g. around calving), even if unlimited access to feed is provided, high-yielding dairy cows may enter a **state of negative energy balance** because the energy demand for maintenance and lactation exceeds the energy intake from feed.

Concern about negative energy balance has been expressed in particular in relation to high-yielding dairy cows fed exclusively with low-energy diets such as grass and other forages. The state of negative energy balance leads to the mobilization of energy reserves (body fat) to be used for maintenance and lactation. Cows experiencing this challenge are sometimes said to be experiencing 'metabolic' hunger; this state results in reduced fertility and milk production, both of which lead to reduced profit.

3.2.2 Prevention of negative energy balance

A common practice to prevent negative energy balance is to increase the energy content of the diet. This can be achieved by increasing the percentage of highly fermentable carbohydrates or by adding fat. However, feeding cows with highly fermentable carbohydrate diets can increase the concentration of lactic acid in the rumen, which is likely to result in acidification (pH < 5.6) of the rumen. If this acidification persists for long periods (>3 h/day), it leads to subacute ruminal acidosis (SARA). SARA reduces feed intake and alters the rumen microbiota and rumen digestion, which may increase the likelihood of development of diarrhoea, laminitis, and liver abscesses, to mention a few. As a result, SARA reduces milk production and has a high economic impact.

As an alternative to carbohydrates, fat addition can be used to provide an extra source of energy in the diet. In high-producing dairy cows, supplementary fat may alleviate the negative energy balance that occurs during early lactation and, consequently, improve fertility and milk yield. The addition of dietary fat soon after calving may also reduce the risk of ketosis and steatosis before peak lactation.

Chronic thirst

Permanent access to fresh and clean water is essential for cows in milk, as a notable quantity of water is secreted in milk. Cows may consume 30–50% of their daily water intake within 1 h after milking. Reported rates of water intake vary from 3 to 15 l/min. Water requirements may depend on several factors, of which physiological status (pregnancy, milk production) and environmental temperature are the most notable. A high-producing dairy cow can drink up to three times the volume of its production in milk. This means that a cow producing 40 litres of milk may drink up to 120 litres of water a day. These requirements can be even higher in the event of heat stress (THI >75; see section 4.2).

3.2.3 Obesity

However, if the addition of fat to the diet leads to excessive deposition of body fat (obesity), it can result, for example, in a fatty liver, impairing animal health and welfare. After calving, the liver plays a key role in making energy available for lactation. A fatty liver likely triggers clinical ketosis, thus reducing the availability of energy for normal functioning in a period of high energy demand. Furthermore, fat deposition through-out the body increases the cow's body condition score (BCS); if a certain threshold BCS is exceeded at calving, this can compromise the health of the cow as well as the survival of the calf. A BCS above 3.5 (out of 5) at calving, compared with a BCS of 3, is associated with a reduction in early lactation, dry matter intake, an increase in metabolic disorders, and a greater risk of mastitis, ketosis, and milk fever after calving.

3.3 Impact of feeding behaviour on animal welfare and productivity

Production and efficiency are affected by the amount of feed eaten but also by the way the feed is consumed (Figure 3.1). Among the main aspects related to feeding that affect productivity are **feed quantity and quality and feeding behaviour**. The nutritional requirements of a cow are highly dependent on the level of milk production. For instance, in a high-producing dairy cow, the nutritional requirements are likely to be high, and the feed should be able to provide sufficient amounts of the necessary nutrients (proteins, carbohydrates, vitamins, etc.) to fulfil the animal's demands. In essence, both the quantity and the quality of feed should be tailored to the nutritional requirements of the cow.

In addition to providing enough nutrients to the cow in the feed, suitable nutrition is also determined by **the way the feed is consumed**. The way cows eat, or their feeding behaviour, can be notably affected by their social behaviour and health status. For instance, hierarchy plays a key role in the access of each animal to resources that are limited (such as feed), as mentioned in section 3.1. Painful conditions such as lameness may reduce the capacity of cows to move, including movements to the feeder, and therefore affect the way they eat. Changes in feeding behaviour have an impact on milk production. Furthermore, the correlation between milk production (kg/day) and feeding behaviour (time spent eating) is stronger than the relationship between milk production and

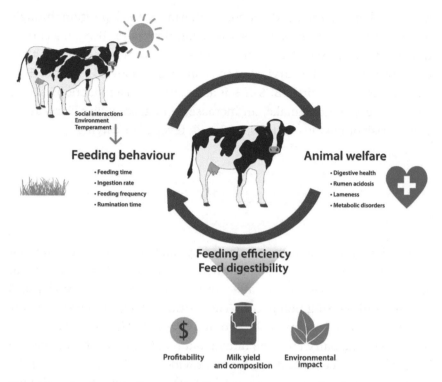

Figure 3.1 Reciprocal effects of feeding behaviour and animal welfare that ultimately influence productivity and profitability (adapted, with permission, from Llonch et al., 2018).

feed intake. Feeding behaviour can affect productivity in various ways. First, an increase in the time spent eating facilitates chewing, which reduces feed particle size and increases digestibility. Second, a longer feeding time increases the production of saliva, which acts as a buffer over the surface of the rumen, decreasing acidity. Sorting behaviour (see section 3.5) has also been identified to potentially impact productivity. Dairy cows receiving a mixed ration typically select in favour of short and fine particles of feed and against longer pieces of forage. This pattern may result in an imbalanced nutrient intake in relation to the formulated diet, resulting in negative consequences for efficiency and production.

In addition to feed intake and feeding behaviour, **rumination** is also a key trait for proper digestive functioning in cattle. Rumination aims to make feed (especially forage) more accessible for microorganisms that facilitate the fermentation of fibre and increase its digestibility. Rumination time also has an impact on milk production, probably as a result of the positive association between rumination and the time cows spend lying down. Rumination time is positively correlated with milk production during the first weeks of lactation.

3.4 Feeding behaviour indicators

Feeding is associated with the metabolic and health status of cows; for this reason, feeding behaviour has been used as a proxy for animal fitness. One of the first signs that can be identified in unfit animals is that they change their feeding pattern. **This change is not only about the quantity of feed they ingest but also about how they eat**. For instance, the average duration of meals can predict changes in rumination during ruminal acidosis. Therefore, feed intake and feeding behaviour can provide key information about the welfare status of a cow. Whereas feed intake considers the quantity of feed ingested during meals, usually through the dry portion of feed, feeding behaviour describes the temporal distribution of feed intake. Measurements commonly used to describe feeding behaviour include the frequency and duration of meals. However, feeding behaviour can also be assessed using a variety of additional variables. In confined animals, the variables that are commonly used to monitor feeding include:

- the quantity of dry matter intake (DMI; kg/day)
- average intake per visit to the feeder (kg/visit)
- number of visits to the feeder (visits/day)
- time spent at the feeder (min/day)
- average time per visit to the feeder (min/visit)
- feeding rate (g/min).

These measures may not be applicable for the assessment of feeding in cattle at pasture. For animals at pasture, the reference variable to assess feeding is the estimated DMI, which can be calculated on the basis of time spent grazing, the biting rate, and the bite size, using the following equation.

$$\text{Pasture DMI} = \text{grazing time} \times \text{biting rate} \times \text{bite size}$$

3.5 Sorting behaviour

Another measure that can be used to describe the feeding behaviour of cows is sorting behaviour. Dairy cattle selectively consume (sort for) the shorter, concentrated particles in their total mixed ration, while selectively refusing (sort against) the longer forage particles. This behaviour can be assessed by comparing the proportions and weight of constituents of the diet offered and the orts (the feed left uneaten). Smaller particles, such as concentrate or pellets, can be consumed at a higher rate than longer particles, such as long, fibrous forages. The importance of sorting behaviour lies in its association with digestion efficiency and production. Smaller particles are more accessible to the ruminal microflora and are readily digestible, which increases the risk of cattle developing ruminal acidosis.

In recent years, numerous tools, such as pedometers or electronic collars, have been developed to automatically monitor behaviour in cows. Accelerometers are used to monitor the movements of cows to estimate their activity and feeding behaviour. An alternative to accelerometers is the 'jaw movement' recorder (IGER Behaviour Recorder), which can be used to monitor feeding behaviour in grazing cattle through a time-stamped record of bites and chews.

'Important aspects to safeguard welfare in dairy cows include freedom from hunger and thirst.'

3.6 Recommendations

3.6.1 Access to water

Cows must be provided with free access to clean, fresh water. The length of water troughs should be 6 cm per cow (10 cm per cow under heat-stress conditions) and their optimal height is 70–80 cm. At least two drinkers are needed for each group of cows. Drinkers should be situated in locations where cows have more motivation to drink, for example, where they exit the milking parlour. Water flow should not be less than 12 l/min, especially in drinker bowls and in latitudes where heat stress is likely (Figure 3.2).

The temperature of drinking water can have an effect on cows' water intake (Figure 3.3). Given a choice of water temperature, cows prefer to drink water at a moderate temperature (approximately 15–25°C) rather than very cold or warm water. In cold conditions, water intake can be severely decreased, consequently reducing milk production.

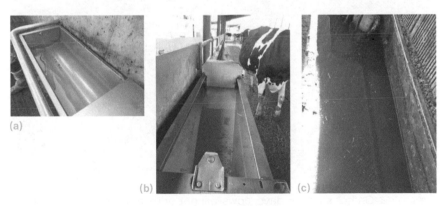

(a)

(b)

(c)

Figure 3.2 Cleanliness of drinkers: (a) drinker and water clean; (b) drinker dirty, but water fresh and clean; (c) drinker and water dirty.

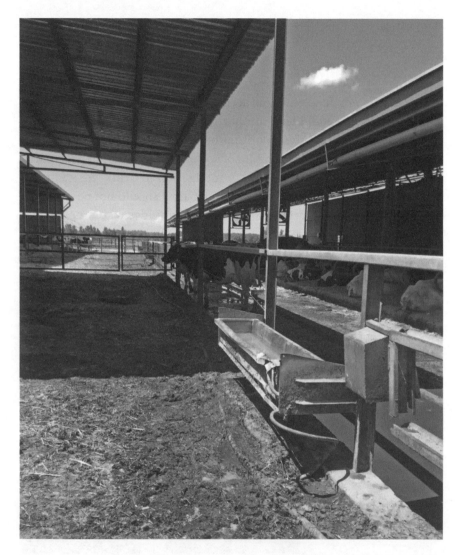

Figure 3.3 On hot summer days, cows will not drink from drinkers located in direct sunlight, as the temperature of the water quickly increases.

3.6.2 Access to feed

Feeding should guarantee that animals receive all nutrients to meet their demand. This entails not only providing enough feed but also that the nutritional quality of the diet matches the animals' requirements. In cases where the energy need is higher than the nutrient intake, the diet should be supplemented with a higher proportion of starch or fat, or both.

A feeding space of at least 60 cm per dairy cow is recommended, whereas for dry cows more space (0.75–0.80 m) should be provided. Besides space availability, the design of the feed bunk can also influence dominance behaviour, and it should guarantee that all animals can have access to feed at the same time. If headlocks are present, there should be as many as the number of cows in the barn. In addition, to avoid competition for access to feed, the feeding management can stimulate feeding at multiple times through the day by, for instance, regularly bringing the feed closer to the cows.

To prevent ruminal acidosis, rations must contain at a minimum ~30% of neutral detergent fibre and have a food particle size no smaller than ~2.8 mm. Slow-degradation cereals such as corn and sorghum should be used to minimize the risk of ruminal acidosis. The change of forage to concentrate in the diet should be carried out gradually over a period of at least 15 days. Ruminal acidosis can also be mitigated by using dietary strategies such as the inclusion of additives with a buffer capacity and antioxidants.

Bibliography

Aikman, P.C., Reynolds, C.K. and Beever, D.E. (2008) Diet digestibility, rate of passage, and eating and rumination behavior of Jersey and Holstein cows. *Journal of Dairy Science* 91, 1103–1114.

Bach, A., Dinarés, M., Devant, M. and Carré, X. (2007) Associations between lameness and production, feeding and milking attendance of Holstein cows milked with an automatic milking system. *Journal of Dairy Research* 74, 40–46.

Bareille, N., Beaudeau, F., Billon, S., Robert, A. and Faverdin, P. (2003) Effects of health disorders on feed intake and milk production in dairy cows. *Livestock Production Science* 83, 53–62.

Bargo, F., Muller, L.D., Kolver, E.S. and Delahoy, J.E. (2003) Invited review: Production and digestion of supplemented dairy cows on pasture. *Journal of Dairy Science* 86, 1–42.

Beauchemin, K.A. (1991) Ingestion and mastication of feed by dairy cattle. *Veterinary Clinics of North America: Food Animal Practice* 7, 439–463.

Beauchemin K.A. (2018) Invited review: Current perspectives on eating and rumination activity in dairy cows. *Journal of Dairy Science* 101, 4762–4784.

Chapinal, N., Veira, D.M., Weary, D.M. and von Keyserlingk, M.A.G (2007) Technical note: Validation of a system for monitoring and feeding single drinking behavior and intake in group-housed cattle. *Journal of Dairy Science* 90, 5732–5736.

Colucci, P.E., Chase, L.E. and Van Soest, P.J. (1982) Feed intake, apparent diet digestibility, and rate of particulate passage in dairy cattle. *Journal of Dairy Science* 65, 1445–1456.

DeVries, T.J., Beauchemin, K.A., Dohme, F. and Schwartzkopf-Genswein, K.S. (2009) Repeated ruminal acidosis challenges in lactating dairy cows at high and low risk for developing acidosis: feeding, ruminating, and lying behavior. *Journal of Dairy Science* 92, 5067–5078.

DeVries, T.J., Beauchemin, K.A. and von Keyserlingk, M.A.G. (2007) Dietary forage concentration affects the feed sorting behavior of lactating dairy cows. *Journal of Dairy Science* 90, 5572–5579.

DeVries, T.J., von Keyserlingk, M.A.G. and Weary, D.M. (2004) Effect of feeding space on the inter-cow distance, aggression, and feeding behaviour of free-stall housed lactating dairy cows. *Journal of Dairy Science* 87, 1432–1438.

Gillund, P., Reksen, O., Grohn, Y.T. and Karlberg, K. (2001). Body condition related to ketosis and reproductive performance in Norwegian dairy cows. *Journal of Dairy Science* 84, 1390–1396.

Ginane, C., Bonnet, M., Baumont, R. and Revell, D.K. (2015) Feeding behaviour in ruminants: a consequence of interactions between a reward system and the regulation of metabolic homeostasis. *Animal Production Science* 55, 247–260.

González, L.A., Tolkamp, B.J., Coffey, M.P., Ferret, A. and Kyriazakis, I. (2008) Changes in feeding behavior as possible indicators for the automatic monitoring of health disorders in dairy cows. *Journal of Dairy Science* 91, 1017–1028.

Greter, A.M. and DeVries, T.J. (2011) Effect of feeding amount on the feeding and sorting behaviour of lactating dairy cattle. *Canadian Journal of Animal Science* 91, 47–54.

Llonch, P., Mainau, E., Ipharraguerre, I.R., Bargo, F., Tedó, G., Blanch, M. and Manteca, X. (2018) Chicken or the egg: the reciprocal association between feeding behavior and animal welfare and their impact on productivity in dairy cows. *Frontiers in Veterinary Science* 5, 305.

Llonch, P., Somarriba, M., Duthie, C.A., Troy, S., Roehe, R. and Rooke, J. (2018) Temperament and dominance relate to feeding behaviour and activity in beef cattle: implications for performance and methane emissions. *Animal* 12, 2639–2648.

Macmillan, K., Gao, X. and Oba, M. (2017) Increased feeding frequency increased milk fat yield and may reduce the severity of subacute ruminal acidosis in higher-risk cows. *Journal of Dairy Science* 100, 1045–1054.

Milam, K.Z., Coppock, C.E., West, J.W., Lanham, J.K., Nave, D.H., Labore, J.M., Stermer, R.A. and Brasington, C.F. (1986) Effects of drinking water temperature on production in lactating Holstein cows in summer. *Journal of Dairy Science* 69, 1013–1019.

Norring, M., Häggman, J., Simojoki, H., Tamminen, P., Winckler, C. and Pastell, M. (2014) Short communication: Lameness impairs feeding behaviour of dairy cows. *Journal of Dairy Science* 97, 4317–4321.

Owens, F.N., Secrist, D.S., Hill, W.J. and Gill, D.R. (1998) Acidosis in cattle: a review. *Journal of Dairy Science* 76, 275–286.

Plaizier, J.C., Krause, D.O., Gozho, G.N. and McBride, B.W. (2008) Subacute ruminal acidosis in dairy cows: the physiological causes, incidence and consequences. *Veterinary Journal* 176, 21–31.

Polsky, L. and von Keyserlingk, M.A.G. (2017) Invited review: Effects of heat stress on dairy cattle welfare. *Journal of Dairy Science* 100, 8645–8657.

Rioja-Lang, F.C., Roberts, D.J., Healy, S.D., Lawrence, A.B. and Haskell, M.J. (2012) Dairy cow feeding space requirements assessed in a Y-maze choice test. *Journal of Dairy Science* 95, 3954–3960.

Roche, J.R., Friggens, N.C., Kay, J.K., Fisher, M.W., Stafford, K.J. and Berry, D.P. (2009) Invited review: Body condition score and its association with dairy cow productivity, health, and welfare. *Journal of Dairy Science* 92, 5769–5801.

Shabi, Z., Murphy, M.R. and Moallem, U. (2005) Within-day feeding behavior of lactating dairy cows measured using a real-time control system. *Journal of Dairy Science* 88, 1848–1854.

Soriani, N., Trevisi, E. and Calamari, L. (2012) Relationships between rumination time, metabolic conditions, and health status in dairy cows during the transition period. *Journal of Dairy Science* 90, 4544–4554.

Sova, A.D., LeBlanc, S.J., McBride, B.W. and DeVries, T.J. (2013) Associations between herd-level feeding management practices, feed sorting, and milk production in freestall dairy farms. *Journal of Dairy Science* 96, 4759–4770.

Von Keyserlingk, M.A.G. and Weary, D.M. (2010) Review: Feeding behaviour of dairy cattle: measures and applications. *Canadian Journal of Animal Science* 90, 303–309.

Weary, D.M., Huzzey, J.M. and von Keyserlingk, M.A.G. (2009) Board-invited review: Using behavior to predict and identify ill health in animals. *Journal of Dairy Science* 87, 770–777.

CHAPTER 4

Welfare issues related to housing

Welfare issues related to the housing of dairy cattle take into consideration the animals' comfort around resting and their thermal comfort. **Comfort around resting** focuses on lying behaviour, which is a high-priority behaviour for dairy cows. Housing has a substantial effect on lying behaviour, which in turn impacts the health and performance of dairy cattle. Each housing system has its own advantages and disadvantages in terms of animal welfare. **Thermal comfort**, which focuses on heat stress, is one of the greatest challenges faced by dairy farmers in many regions of the world. High temperatures depress the feed intake, milk production, and reproductive performance of cows.

4.1 Lying behaviour

4.1.1 Importance of lying behaviour

Dairy cows are highly motivated to lie down for approximately 10–12 h/day. Lying is a high-priority behaviour, and is prioritized even higher than eating and social contact when opportunities to perform these behaviours are restricted. Having enough time for lying is important, as inadequate lying time can affect both the production and welfare of dairy cows. A cow that is lying is more likely to ruminate and produce saliva than a standing cow, thus reducing its risk of ruminal acidosis. A lying cow also has a higher rate of blood diffusion through the udder (~ 5 l/min) compared with a standing animal (~ 3 l/min). This improves udder function and milk production. When a cow spends too much time standing, the pressure inside the claw capsule increases, resulting in hypoxia (restricted oxygen supply) and ischaemia (restricted blood flow), and thus increasing the risk of lameness. Furthermore, competition for a comfortable resting place can trigger social conflicts among cows, increasing the likelihood of chronic stress reactions, which predispose herds to diseases and reproductive problems.

> *'Ensuring adequate resting behaviour positively affects both production and welfare in dairy cows.'*

Several behavioural indicators are used to evaluate cows' comfort around resting, such as the time spent lying down, the frequency of bouts of lying, and the duration of individual bouts. Cows on comfortable flooring lie down for longer overall but the duration of each lying bout is shorter, meaning that the cows stand up more frequently and remain standing for shorter periods of time. Cows prefer to remain standing rather than experience the pain associated with a lying or rising movement when they are housed on rough resting surfaces. Two additional behavioural indicators that may suggest discomfort around resting are the number of cows lying partially or totally out of the resting area (Figure 4.1) and an increase in the number of cows 'perching' (Figure 4.2).

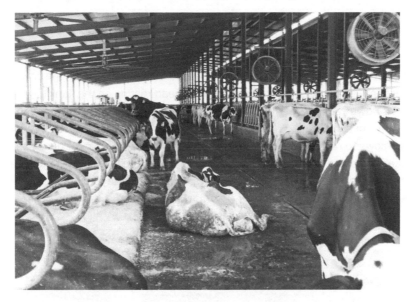

Figure 4.1 Cow lying in the passageway, which is totally out of the resting area.

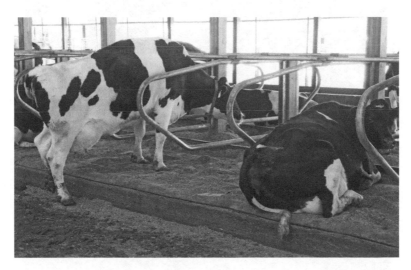

Figure 4.2 Perching behaviour: a cow is standing with the two front feet in the stall and the two hind feet in the corridor.

Sleep is important for cows too

Adult cattle sleep for about 4 h/day, mainly during the night. Sleep, especially REM (rapid eye movement) sleep, occurs most often when the cow is resting with the neck relaxed and with the head resting on the flank (Figure 4.3). Cows that are well adapted to their surroundings rarely engage in sleep while standing. A decrease in lying time reduces the possibility for the cows to rest and sleep. A reduction in lying time due to poor housing is likely to have a more severe effect on animal welfare if it reduces the time spent sleeping. Lack of sleep can alter the endocrine system, increase energy expenditure, and impair the immune function.

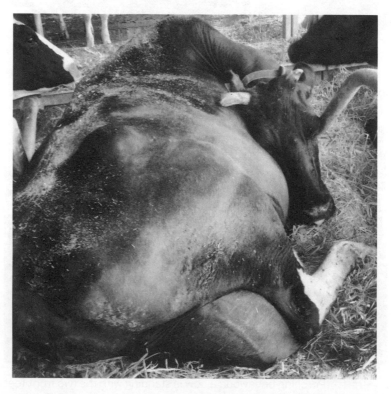

Figure 4.3 Dairy cow in a lying posture, which is often associated with sleep.

4.1.2 Main welfare problems related to housing

Housing has a substantial impact on the lying behaviour, overall health, and performance of dairy cattle. There is no single best housing system for lactating cows in terms of animal welfare, and the animals' management has a big impact and probably makes the difference. Loose housing of cows in stalls is the most common type of housing used in intensive dairy farming. Stalls can vary in terms of their design, type of bedding, and floor quality. The dimensions of stalls are not always adjusted to the body size of the cows. Inappropriate stall dimensions lead to an increase in the number of cows perching inside the stall and lying outside the lying area. Uncomfortable stalls reduce the cows' lying time due to their inability to adopt certain resting postures. This will alter their sleep patterns and thereby have a negative impact on their performance (Figure 4.4). Lying down and rising movements are easier for the cows when the stalls are correctly designed and provide a soft bedding area. Soft flooring reduces the incidence of swelling of the front knees, which occurs because cows place weight on their front knees when they get up and lie down. The hardness of the lying surface and the use of concrete, abrasive, and slippery flooring increase the risk of injuries and lameness.

Loose housing systems with deep bedding, including straw or compost, are increasing in popularity in Europe (Figure 4.5). Dairy cows have a clear preference for standing and lying in a straw-yard system than in a stall system, and the longest durations of lying time are reported on deep-bedded systems. Behavioural indicators related to resting suggest that cows are more comfortable in bedded pack barns than in stalls. The incidence of injuries to both the front and hind legs is also reduced in deep-litter systems. However, deep-litter systems require intensive labour and have higher costs related to the bedding material. If they are not correctly managed, deep-litter systems can trigger problems related to the hygiene of the animals. Cows housed in deep-bedding systems tend to be dirtier, increasing the risk of mastitis. Cows avoid manure-covered floors in preference for floors that are dry, wet or

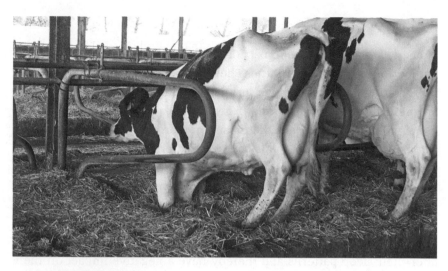

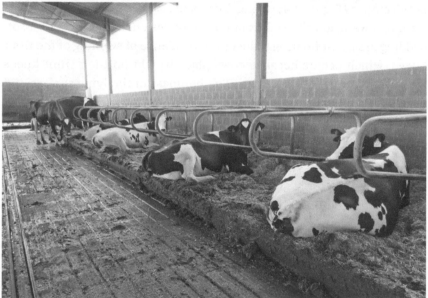

Figure 4.4 (Top) The head and body of a cow are thrust forward 0.6–0.7 m while the cow is lying down or rising. (Bottom) A poorly designed cubicle (without a lunge zone) does not permit normal lying down and rising behaviour, and reduces comfort at resting.

consist of earth. Good hygiene is essential to reduce the incidence of infectious diseases, such as mastitis, in these systems. Moreover, excessive manure on the floor softens the hooves, which are then more prone to mechanical damage. The interdigital skin becomes softer because of the accumulated manure, which exposes the deeper tissues to microorganisms and predisposes these areas to infectious diseases. The quality of the bedding area and its management are very important to prevent diseases related to environmental pathogens.

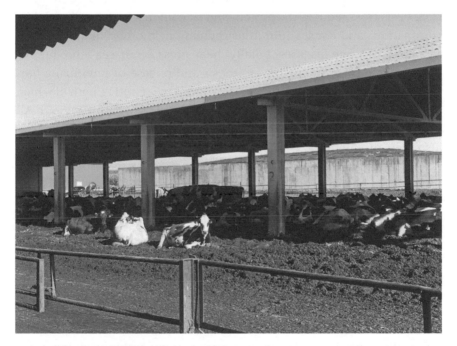

Figure 4.5 Compost bedding pack barn.

4.2 Thermal stress

4.2.1 Economic impact of heat stress

Heat stress is a major factor that reduces milk production in dairy cows. Up to 10% of the variability in milk production has been attributed to the effect of climatic factors such as temperature. The decrease in milk production under heat-stress situations is directly linked to a reduction in feed intake, while the energy needs of the animal increase. In addition, heat stress reduces the protein and fat contents in the milk, inhibits rumination, and causes immunosuppression, thereby increasing the incidence of some diseases. Finally, heat stress decreases reproductive performance by reducing the synthesis and release of luteinizing hormone (LH) and gonadotropin-releasing hormone (GnRH), both of which are essential for ovulation and the expression of oestrous behaviour. All of these effects of heat stress impact not only the welfare of cows but also their productivity, which is directly associated with the economic return for the farmer.

4.2.2 What does thermal stress mean?

The feeling of warmth, the so-called effective temperature, depends on the ambient temperature and also on other environmental variables. It results from the interaction of several factors, especially temperature, relative humidity, ventilation, and solar radiation. The temperature and humidity index (THI) is often used in dairy cows to estimate the effective temperature based, as the name suggests, upon ambient temperature and relative humidity records. Traditionally, it has been considered that when the THI exceeds a value of 72 (e.g. 25°C temperature and 50% humidity), cows begin to suffer heat stress. However, recent studies suggest that some cows, especially highly productive ones, are negatively affected by THI values as low as 68. In any case, the combination of high ambient temperature and high relative humidity is always problematic.

'Milk yield declines by 0.2 kg per cow and day per each unit increase of THI when this index exceeds 72.'

Thermal stress in dairy cows varies according to many variables, including their breed, milk production level, the quantity and quality of their feed, their health status, and their level of hydration, which can intensify the effects of high temperatures. For example, a high-producing cow (> 30 kg of milk/day) generates 48 % more heat than a dry cow, and therefore is at a higher risk of suffering heat stress. Cows at the beginning of lactation are also more likely to suffer heat stress. The dramatic increase in heat production by these animals is due to increases in both milk production and feed ingestion.

4.2.3 How does heat stress affect high yield dairy cows?

Dairy cows have different physiological and behavioural mechanisms to adapt to hot environments. Physiological mechanisms include an increase in the respiratory rate and panting, and, to a lower extent, sweating. At the hormonal level, thermal stress activates the stress response, with the consequent release of glucocorticoids. High levels of glucocorticoids result in a decrease in both the ingestion of dry matter and the efficiency of the conversion of feed into milk. In addition, high levels of glucocorticoids compromise the function of the immune system and therefore increase susceptibility to infectious diseases.

Under heat-stress conditions, dairy cows increase the time they spend standing and decrease the time they spend resting. Standing allows cows to maximize the body surface area in contact with air and so increase heat dissipation. However, the alteration of resting behaviour can have serious consequences for production and the appearance of lameness.

High temperatures are associated with a reduction in dry matter intake, which is reflected in a considerable reduction in the cows' body condition.

Dairy cows show signs of severe dehydration at water loss levels equivalent to more than 10% of body weight. Water consumption increases more than 1 litre for every 1°C increase in ambient temperature. Hyperthermia (increase of body temperature) and dehydration have been associated with an increase in neuromuscular fatigue and incoordination of movement in animals. This means that in hot climates the risk of injury due to trauma can increase.

4.2.4 Recommendations to reduce heat stress

The effect of heat stress on dairy production should be minimized by combining the most cost-effective strategies that are feasible in terms of handling and additional management. Strategies to tackle heat stress include the provision of shade for the animals, optimization of water intake, the use of water-spray systems and ventilation, and modifications of the diet.

It is essential that cows have access to clean, fresh drinking water. When using long drinkers, it is recommended that the total length of the drinking trough be equivalent to at least 6 cm per cow. Under heat-stress conditions, it is recommended to increase this length to 10 cm per cow. Ideally, there should be at least two drinkers per pen.

Heat dissipation mostly depends upon the evaporation of water from the skin and upper airways. At ambient temperatures above 25°C, heat loss by dissipation is markedly reduced. Therefore, maintaining productivity in warm climates will mostly depend on improving heat dissipation by modification of the environmental heat load (e.g. increasing ventilation) and increasing heat loss from the surface of the animals.

It is estimated that digestion processes generate an increase of up to 20% of heat production from basal levels. Consequently, and as mentioned, one of the main effects of high temperatures is a reduction in feed intake. Some feeding strategies to reduce thermal stress are:

Cows should take several showers a day

The only way to guarantee a positive effect on productive and reproductive indices is to maintain the body temperature of the cows below 39°C, 24 h/day, by means of several daily showers. On very hot days, it is not enough to cool the cows just before milking. One successfully implemented strategy to mitigate heat stress and maintain milk production is to cool cows with six daily 'baths' combining showers with ventilation. Showers take place in the waiting room, not only at each of the two or three daily milkings but also three more times per day, when the cows are brought into the waiting room to be refreshed for 45 min.

- increasing the supply of fat in the diet to increase its energy density
- avoiding an excess of total and degradable protein contents
- optimizing fibre digestibility, especially in high-energy diets
- providing feed at sunrise and sunset.

Sensory additives in the ration – a practical case

In one experiment (Bargo et al., 2014), sensory additives were shown to alleviate the adverse effects of heat stress in 570 milking cows at mid-lactation (with an average milk production of 34.4 kg/day at 194 days of lactation). Half of the cows were given a total mixed ration (TMR) with sensory additives, while the other half continued to eat the routine TMR. During a period of 5 weeks, in which the environmental temperature ranged between 20.4°C and 38.9°C, production data were measured. The cows that received the TMR with sensory additives produced 2 kg of milk/day more than the cows that continued to receive their normal ration. The consumption of dry matter was also higher in the cows that received the sensory additives (+1.2 kg/day). Sensory additives can be a tool to modulate the feeding behaviour of high-producing cows under heat-stress conditions by promoting a higher frequency of visits to the feeder and the consumption of dry matter.

Bibliography

Bargo, F., Muñoz, S., Candelas, M., Vargas, J. and Ipharraguerre, I. (2014) A sensory additive improves performance of dairy cows under heat stress. *Proceedings of the ADSA-ASAS-CSAS Joint Annual Meeting*, Kansas City, MO, USA, Poster 1593.

Berman, A. (1971) Thermoregulation in intensively lactating cows in near natural conditions. *Journal of Physiology* 215, 477–489.

Bewley, J.M., Robertson, L.M. and Eckelkamp, E.A. (2017) A 100-year review: Lactating dairy cattle housing management. *Journal of Dairy Science* 100, 10418–10431.

Cook, N.B. (2019) Optimizing resting behavior in lactating dairy cows through freestall design. *Veterinary Clinics of North America: Food Animal Practice* 35, 93–109.

Cook, N.B. and Nordlund, K.V. (2004) Behavioral needs of the transition cow and considerations for special needs facility design. *Veterinary Clinics of North America: Food Animal Practice* 20, 495–520.

Fernández, A., Mainau, E., Manteca, X., Siurana, A. and Castillejos, L. (2020) Impacts of compost bedded pack barns on the welfare and comfort of dairy cows. *Animals* 10, 431–441.

Flamenbaum, I., Wolfenson, I.D., Mamen, M. and Berman, A. (1986) Cooling dairy cattle by a combination of sprinkling and forced ventilation and its implementation in the shelter system. *Journal of Dairy Science*, 69, 3140–3147.

Fregonesi, J.A. and Leaver, J.D. (2001) Behaviour, performance and health indicators of welfare for dairy cows housed in strawyard or cubicle systems. *Livestock Production Science* 68, 205–216.

Haskell, M.J., Rennie, L.J., Bowell, V.A., Bell, M.J. and Lawrence, A.B. (2006) Housing system, milk production, and zero-grazing effects on lameness and leg injury in dairy cows. *Journal of Dairy Science* 89, 4259–4266.

Herbut, P., Angrecka, S. and Walczak, J. (2018) Environmental parameters to assessing of heat stress in dairy cattle – a review. *International Journal of Biometeorology* 62, 2089–2097.

Polsky, L. and von Keyserlingk, M.A.G. (2017) Invited review: Effects of heat stress on dairy cattle welfare. *Journal of Dairy Science* 100, 8645–8657.

Ravagnolo, O. and Misztal, I. (2000) Genetic component of heat stress in dairy cattle, parameter estimation. *Journal of Dairy Science* 83, 2126–2130.

Temple, D., Bargo, F., Mainau, E., Ipharraguerre, I. and Manteca, X. (2015) Heat stress and efficiency in dairy milk production: a practical approach. Fact Sheet 12. *Farm Animal Welfare Education Centre*, Barcelona, Spain. Available at: https://www.fawec.org/en/technical-documents-cattle/131-heat-stress-and-efficiency-in-dairy-milk-production-a-practical-approach (accessed 22 November 2021).

Temple, D., Bargo, F., Mainau, E., Ipharraguerre, I. and Manteca, X. (2016) Lying behaviour and performances in dairy cattle – practical case. Fact Sheet 15. *Farm Animal Welfare Education Centre*, Barcelona, Spain. Available at: https://www.fawec.org/en/technical-documents-cattle/196-lying-performance-dairy-cattle (accessed 22 November 2021).

West, J.W. (2003) Effects of heat-stress on production in dairy cattle. *Journal of Dairy Science*, 86, 2131–2144.

Whitaker, D.A., Kelly, J.M. and Smith, S. (2000) Disposal and disease rates in 340 British dairy herds. *Veterinary Record* 146, 363–367.

CHAPTER 5

Welfare issues related to health

Health is an important component of animal welfare and must be considered when assessing welfare. Disease and injuries may have a negative effect on the emotional state of an animal (through the pain and distress they cause) and may also interfere with its normal behaviour. Animals must be protected from pain, injury, and disease by prevention, and rapid diagnosis and treatment.

5.1 General aspects of health

If animals are healthy, it does not mean that other aspects of their welfare are always satisfactory. However, animals that are cared for in accordance with acceptable welfare standards are more likely to be healthy and, conversely, animals kept in poor welfare conditions are often at a greater risk of disease. Improving health can improve growth, reproduction, and productivity.

> *'Welfare is not synonymous with health. While good health is critical to welfare, the concept of welfare is much broader and encompasses other aspects as well.'*

Disease has several negative effects on animal welfare and behaviour.

- **Pain and suffering**. Some diseases cause the animal to experience unpleasant sensory and/or emotional states, associated with actual or potential tissue damage (e.g. lameness, mastitis, dystocia).
- **Sickness behaviour**. When an animal becomes sick due to an infection or injury, its immune system initiates strategic behavioural changes in order to facilitate the conservation of energy. Sickness behaviour is characterized by reduced feed intake, apathy, weakness, and lethargy. Sickness behaviour is a well-organized adaptive response of the animal to enhance its resistance against, and recovery from, disease.
- Diseased animals might also experience **other negative emotional states**, such as fear (because of disorientation or reduced ability to respond to perceived danger) and distress (e.g. hypoxia in diseases that impair the supply of oxygen to the body).
- Some diseases can cause **discomfort** (e.g. skin diseases such as mite infestation) or **prolonged immobility** (e.g. lameness).

5.1.1 Identification of sick dairy cows

In recent years, the identification of sick dairy cows in an early state of disease by observing the behaviour of individual cows has become more and more important. The standard approach for this task is direct visual observation, which traditionally serves as a diagnostic tool for farmers and veterinarians. There are several patterns of sickness and/ or pain behaviour that occur in a wide variety of diseases (Table 5.1, Figure 5.1).

Table 5.1 Examples of sickness and/or pain behaviours in dairy cows (adapted from Gleerup et al., 2015 and Dittrich et al., 2019).

Item	Definition
Attention	Quiet or depressed. The cow is not active, does not look at the observer, and may move away from the observer
Head position	At the level of or below the withers of the cow
Head activity	The cow is not active and not ruminating
Ear position	Both ears back or lower than usual. Asymmetrical ear movements
Back position	Slightly or completely arched
Piloerection	Slightly or obviously erect hair coat
Feeding	Reduced feed intake and feeding duration
Physical activity	Reduced or increased duration of lying and standing
Others	Occasional or frequent tooth grinding, vocalization

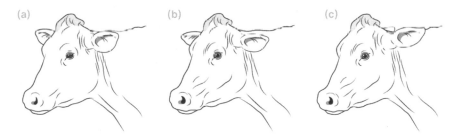

Figure 5.1 Illustrations of the Cow Pain Face. (a) Relaxed cow. (b) Cow in pain with low ears/lamb ears. (c) Cow in pain with ears tense and backwards. (Reprinted from *Applied Animal Behaviour Science*, 171, Karina Bech Gleerup, Pia Haubro Andersen, Lene Munksgaard, Björn Forkman, Pain evaluation in dairy cattle, 25–32, Copyright (2015), with permission from Elsevier).

5.1.2 Hospital pens

Sick or injured cows may have different behavioural priorities and needs from those of healthy cows, and it is recommended to accommodate them in special areas or hospital pens. These areas/pens must have the following features and/or improvements compared with the home pens.

- Smaller group size and more space allowed.
- Low level of competition, with easier access to feed, water, and resting areas.
- Shorter waiting time for milking: lactating sick cows should be milked close to or inside the hospital pen.
- Softer surface and appropriate bedding.
- A shelter that is always accessible.
- Located so as to facilitate the observation, monitoring, and treatment of the cows.

Up to now, there has not been a clear recommendation concerning the use of individual or group hospital pens, or on an optimal stocking density in hospital pens. Sick cows show isolation-seeking behaviour, suggesting that they are more sensitive to regrouping than healthy cows. Regrouping healthy cows with unfamiliar animals leads to increased stress and aggression, as well as to reduced feed intake, rumination, and lying time. However, the possible effects of limited or no social contact on cows housed in individual pens are unknown.

It is recommended to move cows with ambulatory difficulties, with conditions such as calving difficulties, injuries, severe lameness, milk fever, or displaced abomasum, to hospital pens. However, for mild illness or injuries (e.g. metritis or moderate lameness), segregation from the home pen may disrupt the social hierarchy of the cows or cause additional stress to the affected animal.

Hospital pens should be occupied only by sick or injured cows. Avoid using these pens for calving and/or dry cows. Mixing sick cows with healthy periparturient cows is not recommended due to the potential for social stress, the risk of transmission of infection, and the different behavioural needs of these groups of cows. For instance, restlessness associated with calving is likely to disturb the convalescent behaviour of sick cows.

If a sick animal that is showing signs of pain or discomfort does not respond to treatment or has an incurable condition, it should be euthanized as soon as possible, and if it cannot be moved or transported without causing more suffering, it should be euthanized where it is.

5.2 Lameness

Lameness is characterized by an abnormal gait that normally results from injury, disease, or dysfunction of one or more feet and/or limbs. Lameness is one of the major animal welfare and economic problems in dairy cattle production. Incidences of lameness as high as 20–35% have been reported in dairy farms. Lameness is a multifactorial disease, and the risk of cows developing lameness is associated with factors such as their management, features of the equipment and facilities in their environment, their nutrition, and genetic selection.

Classification of lameness

Over 90% of all cases of lameness are caused by claw disorders, mainly in the hind limbs. The degree of severity varies based on the type and location of the injury. Several conditions can give rise to lameness, including **infectious** conditions such as digital dermatitis and foot rot, and **non-infectious** conditions such as sole bruises, sole ulcers, white line disease and laminitis. In recent years there has been a general decline in the incidence of non-infectious causes and an increase in infectious causes, particularly digital dermatitis.

5.2.1 Lameness is a painful disease

Dairy producers and veterinarians consider lameness to be one of the most painful conditions in dairy cows. Lame cows suffer from acute and chronic pain, as well as distress. These cows also show increased sensitivity to pain (hyperalgesia) and pain from stimuli that are normally non-painful (allodynia). Hyperalgesia has been observed in cows at the time of detection of lameness and 1 month later, suggesting that these cows are suffering from chronic pain.

Claw lesions are among the major causes of lameness in dairy cows. **Injuries of the claws or the limbs** cause painful bruises, which lead the cow to change its locomotion in an attempt to avoid the pain. **Tissue damage or infections of the claw** can induce **sickness behaviour** (e.g. reduced feed intake and lethargy), as inflammatory cytokines are released in these conditions, but even if an immune reaction is not present, lame cows change their behaviour because of pain.

There are several behavioural indicators of pain caused by lameness (Table 5.2). These behavioural changes are seen not only in severely lame cows but also in moderately lame cows, and can also appear before the cow becomes clinically lame. Lame cows increase their total daily lying time and reduce their daily physical activity (especially walking), as well as spending less time feeding and ruminating. These animals visit the feeder less frequently and eat more at each visit.

In addition, lame cows have physiological changes indicative of stress and pain. These changes include alterations in the heart rate, respiratory rate, temperature, blood pressure, and pupil diameter. Raised levels of cortisol and haptoglobin have been associated with lameness in cows, indicating that lame cows are experiencing stress and pain due to inflammation.

Table 5.2 Behavioural indicators of pain caused by lameness in dairy cattle.

Increased	Additional behavioural signs
Time spent lying down	Lame cows are further back in the milking order
Lying bout duration	Lame cows are more likely to become subordinate and to be subjected to aggressive behaviours from healthy cows
Decreased	Lame cows reduce the use of the automated grooming brush (reduced grooming behaviour)
Physical activity (walking)	Lame cows make fewer visits to the automated milking system
Time spent eating	Lame cows are more reluctant to interact with other cows (reduced social behaviour)
Rumination	
Feeding bouts	

5.2.2 Lameness causes production and economic losses

Lameness is one of the costliest diseases affecting dairy cattle. Lameness is associated with both direct and indirect economic costs (Table 5.3); these costs are usually underestimated by farmers, who thus have a poor perception of its impact on cow welfare and production.

Lame cows produce between 300 and 600 fewer litres of milk per lactation and take 20–40 days longer to get back in calf than cows that are not lame. On average, each case of clinical lameness results in an estimated cost of €450–500.

Lame cows are more prone to develop environmental mastitis (due to the increased time spent lying down) and metabolic disease (especially during the transition period). They also show reduced fertility, as they are unwilling to stand in heat or mount other cows, and can have delayed cycling after calving. Lame cows also lose body condition over time due to changes in their feeding patterns and/or as a consequence of pain affecting feed conversion.

Table 5.3 Main direct and indirect economic costs caused by lameness.

Main direct economic costs	Main indirect economic costs
Reduced milk yield	Increased risk of culling
Increased veterinary costs	Reduced fertility
Discarded milk (during the course of treatment)	Increased risk of further lameness
	Increased risk of secondary disease
	Reduced body condition

'Lame cows have a reduced milk yield for up to 4 months before and 5 months after the clinical evidence of lameness.'

5.2.3 How to identify lameness

Early detection and prompt treatment of lameness reduce the duration and prevalence of lameness and thus improve cow welfare. Many of the early indicators of lameness are subtle and will be seen only by careful inspection of cows while they are walking. The use of **lameness scoring systems** (also known as locomotion scoring systems or LCS) on a regular basis is the most effective means of identifying lameness in cows. LCS describe gait properties to classify the severity of lameness on a numerical scale. There are several valid LCS, using from two-point to nine-point scoring systems. The five-point LCS is one of the most frequently employed methods for lameness detection (Table 5.4).

Cows should be observed under two sets of circumstances.

- Walking on a flat, non-slippery surface for a considerable length of time to assess multiple strides. The presence of manure, or stony or soft tracks, might influence the cows' mobility.
- After milking, as cows walk at their own pace to the paddock, as their locomotion is less likely to be impaired by a swollen udder.

Table 5.4 Example of a lameness scoring system based on a five-point scale (from Sprecher et al., 1997).

Lameness score	Clinical description	Assessment criteria
1	Normal	The cow stands and walks with a level-back posture. Her gait is normal
2	Mildly lame	The cow stands with a level-back posture but develops an arched-back posture while walking. Her gait remains normal
3	Moderately lame	An arched-back posture is evident both while standing and walking. Her gait is affected and is best described as short striding with one or more limbs
4	Lame	An arched-back posture is always evident, and gait is best described as one deliberate step at a time. The cow favours one or more limbs/feet
5	Severely lame	The cow additionally demonstrates an inability or extreme reluctance to bear weight on one or more of her limbs/feet

Generally, LCS include stride length (shortening or lengthening of the stride), steps (asymmetrical gait), the presence of an arched back, and transference of weight to the unaffected limb. Other characteristics that can indicate lameness are stiff joints or reduced step angle, hanging or bobbing of the head during locomotion, and hock posture while standing (Figure 5.2).

In lame and severely lame cows, walking is obviously affected: the cow is unwilling or slow to place one or more feet on the ground, and is likely to be near the back of the herd when walking to be milked. Changes are more difficult to detect in cows with mild or moderate lameness. Apart from alterations in gait presentation and weight bearing, and an arched back, other features such as stiff joints, short steps, and/or one limb moving faster or slower than the others can increase lameness detection.

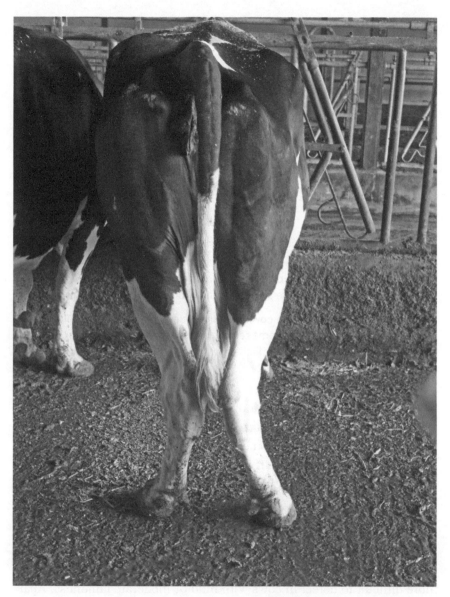

Figure 5.2 The so-called 'cow-hocked' (hocks positioned medially and the hooves of the hind quarters positioned more laterally) stance, which indicates lameness, as the stance is adapted to relieve the pain present in the claw.

Although LCS are the best visual detection systems for lameness, there are some limitations to performing lameness scoring regularly and rigorously. Intra- and inter-observer agreement of LCS is usually moderate (especially in mild cases of lameness), farmers have only a small amount of time to observe lame cows, and many farmers have inadequate knowledge of LCS application. These limitations have encouraged the development of automated systems for lameness detection. Although many prototypes of automatic lameness-detection systems for dairy cattle exist, many of them are still in the research or development phase and have not yet been commercialized. The current systems are mainly able to detect only severe lameness, which can also easily be identified visually.

5.2.4 Prevention of lameness

Lameness control programme and treatment

As the most important risk factor for lameness is inadequate **management** related to poor care and monitoring of foot health, all dairy farmers should implement a lameness prevention programme. This programme should include the following actions.

- Regular weekly locomotion scoring by trained personnel to assess lameness. This facilitates monitoring of the prevalence and severity of lameness, and the identification of ongoing problems and possible causes.
- Foot inspection and trimming should be carried out by a veterinarian or skilled foot trimmer at intervals no greater than 6 months. The discomfort caused by claw lesions can be reduced by corrective trimming techniques and the application of a foot block to the healthy claw.
- Flooring surfaces should be clean and dry, and ideally covered with rubber flooring. Consideration should be given to moving cows to outside areas (when the weather permits). These areas should be

near the milking parlour to reduce the distance the cows are required to walk each day.

- Clinically lame cows should receive prompt veterinary treatment. Pain relief should be provided during and after the treatment of lameness. Pain can be best alleviated by using a **multimodal approach**, including primarily corrective claw trimming and placement of foot blocks, with additional benefits provided by analgesic treatments such as local anaesthetics, non-steroidal anti-inflammatory drugs (NSAIDs), or sedative analgesics. In general, NSAIDs show substantial benefits in models of induced lameness, with improvement of the gait and the pressure placed on the affected foot and claw. However, in field trials, NSAIDs have yielded variable results, with only mild improvements to the locomotion score and nociceptive thresholds.
- Cows that become persistently lame should be culled out of the herd.
- Foot bathing should be used for the prevention of infectious hoof disease in cattle of all ages. It should be applied at least once a week.

Recommendations for an effective footbath

- The footbath should be located on a level floor with a non-slip surface. Ensure that there is easy access to the footbath, with a straight walk through so that cows can follow each other easily. Footbaths should be located at the far end of the lane from the parlour, to avoid cows 'jamming up' at the footbath.
- It should be 3.0–3.7 m long and 0.6 m wide, with a 25 cm high step-in height and sidewalls that slope outwards to reach a width of 0.9 m at a height of 0.9 m above the floor.
- It should be filled to a depth of 10 cm to ensure that the solution washes the interdigital space of cows walking through the bath. The solution should be refreshed every day and also after every 100–300 cow passes.

- Walking the cows through a cleaning bath (containing water or a salt solution) that washes their feet first is recommended because contamination with manure will reduce the activity of the antibacterial agent in the footbath.
- Choose an antibacterial agent with evidence of efficacy for the prevention of new digital dermatitis lesions and foot rot. Traditionally, copper sulphate and formaldehyde were commonly used in footbaths and demonstrated high efficacy. However, in the European Union, the use of both of these agents is illegal: copper sulphate because of environmental concerns, and formaldehyde because it is a carcinogen in humans. Although there are a lot of alternative footbath agents on the market, these products are largely untested and unregulated, thus making it difficult to recommend an effective alternative.

What factors contribute to lameness?

As lameness is a multifactorial disease, several risk factors increase the likelihood of a cow becoming lame. At the same time, these risk factors should be considered in a lameness prevention programme. The main risk factors associated with lameness are shown in Figure 5.3.

Standing and walking on a hard or abrasive floor will negatively impact claw health and locomotion. The use of rubber flooring improves gait properties. For instance, the risk of higher LCS scores is three times greater in cows on a concrete floor compared with a rubber floor. In addition, floors that are wet or covered in slurry increase the risk of lameness for two reasons: (1) coating of the legs with manure enhances the growth of pathogenic organisms capable of invading the digital skin and makes the hooves softer, thus contributing to digital dermatitis and infectious lameness; and (2) the presence of manure on the floors makes them more slippery, thus increasing the incidence of lameness.

The level of comfort of the cows' lying surface might influence the severity of hock lesions (swellings and injuries) as well as increase the

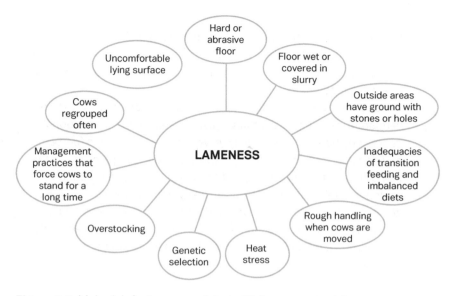

Figure 5.3 Main risk factors associated with lameness in dairy cows.

risk of lameness. Dairy cows have been reported to prefer lying down on softer surfaces. For instance, more discomfort in lying down and a higher incidence of clinical lameness have been observed in cows lying on rubber mats, compared with those on sand.

Rough handling when cows are moved to the milking parlour greatly contributes to the development of severe lameness due to slips. It is important to avoid pushing and hitting the cows when they are moved to the milking parlour. Handlers should walk slowly and follow the recommended position for driving cows (see section 6.3).

Heat stress is considered a risk factor for lameness, but whether this association is a consequence of increased standing time or of alterations in nutrient metabolism caused by a decrease in dry matter intake under heat stress conditions is not known. Finally, genetic selection for high milk yield with insufficient emphasis on other traits related to fitness increases the risk of lameness. Poor hoof and leg conformation can lead to misshapen hooves that are weak and prone to injury.

5.3 Mastitis

Mastitis is an infection of the mammary gland caused by a number of different bacteria. Mastitis is one of the major animal welfare and economic problems in dairy cattle production. Although in recent years there has been a general decline in the incidence of mastitis, **high incidences** of 25–45% are still being reported. Mastitis is a **multifactorial** disease in which the environment, the pathogens, and the host (cow) interact with each other.

Classification of mastitis

Mastitis is generally classified as **clinical** or **subclinical** depending on the degree of inflammation in the mammary gland. Bacterial infections are the most common causes of inflammation of the mammary gland.

Cows with **clinical mastitis** usually have apparent inflammation of the udder, and their milk may contain flakes or blood. Clinical mastitis is classified as mild, moderate, or severe. Cows with clinical mastitis may also be systemically affected and have fever, dehydration, and refuse to eat.

Cows with **subclinical mastitis** do not show visible udder inflammation and can be diagnosed by means of a somatic cell count (SCC) or the California Mastitis Test. The majority of somatic cells are leukocytes (white blood cells), which become present in milk usually as an immune response to mastitis caused by a pathogen.

Mastitis pathogens are classified as either **contagious or environmental**.

Contagious pathogens, such as *Staphylococcus aureus*, *Streptococcus dysgalactiae*, and *Streptococcus agalactiae*, survive within the host and typically spread from cow to cow during milking. In contrast, environmental pathogens, such as *Escherichia coli*, *Streptococcus uberis*, *Enterococcus faecalis*, and *Klebsiella* spp., are opportunistic invaders of the mammary gland and can be found in a variety of substrates, such as litter and manure.

5.3.1 Mastitis causes production and economic losses

Mastitis is one of the costliest diseases affecting dairy cattle. Mastitis is associated with both direct and indirect economic costs, which are usually underestimated by farmers (Table 5.5).

Table 5.5 Main direct and indirect economic costs caused by mastitis.

Main direct economic costs	Main indirect economic costs
Reduced milk yield	Increased risk of culling
Poor-quality milk	Reduced fertility
Increased veterinary costs	
Discarded milk (during the course of treatment)	
Somatic cell count (SCC) penalties	

On average, each case of clinical mastitis causes an estimated loss of around €200. The cost of subclinical mastitis depends on the number of cows with an increased SCC and is mainly attributed to losses in milk production.

5.3.2 Mastitis is a painful disease

Dairy producers and veterinarians consider cases of severe mastitis to be among the most painful conditions in dairy cows. However, it is well known that cows can also experience pain in cases of mild or moderate mastitis. Even subclinical mastitis is accompanied by increased levels of bradykinin, a peptide that mediates the inflammation related to mastitis.

'All clinical mastitis, whether severe or mild, cause pain.'

Cows with mastitis show several signs of **sickness behaviour**, such as reduced feed intake and lethargy. As we stated in section 5.1, sickness behaviour is an adaptive response of the animal to enhance its disease resistance and recovery from disease. Pain caused by mastitis may modify the expression of sickness behaviour. In particular, although lying time is usually increased during illness and is thought to help the animal conserve energy, cows with mastitis show a reduction in lying time because of udder pain, and this has important negative effects on their welfare and production. Some studies report pronounced changes in the laterality of lying behaviour, with cows decreasing the time spent lying on the same side as the affected udder quarter.

Several further behavioural and physiological indicators of udder pain have been defined (Table 5.6). Increased restlessness, such as a higher frequency of kicking and stepping, during milking has been observed for at least 3 days after mastitis detection. The distance between the hocks when the cow is standing is wider in cows with mastitis than in

Table 5.6 Indicators of pain caused by mastitis in dairy cattle.

Behavioural indicators	Physiological and production indicators
Increased	Increased
Restlessness during milking	Heart and respiratory rate
Hock-to-hock distance when standing	Rectal temperature
	Acute phase proteins
Decreased	Decreased
Time spent lying down	Milk yield and quality
Time spent eating	Dry matter intake
Rumination	
Self-grooming	

healthy cows, suggesting that there is a change in the hind leg stance of the cows as a result of the inflamed udder.

Other animal-based indicators such as an increase in the time cows take to enter the milking area, stopping and turning around, kicking off teat cups, increased residual milk, evidence of teat injuries, and increased avoidance of humans could indicate problems with the maintenance of milking equipment or an inadequate milking procedure that is causing udder pain and increasing the risk of mastitis.

Besides reducing rumination, mastitis may also reduce the motility of the rumen, leading to disruption of the microbial degradation of ingested feed.

In terms of physiological indicators, the concentrations of acute phase proteins (APPs) such as serum amyloid A and haptoglobin rapidly increase in the serum and milk of cows with mastitis. APPs have been shown to be good indicators of infection, stress, inflammation, and pain associated with mastitis.

Severe cases of mastitis lead to hyperalgesia (increased pain sensitivity) and allodynia (a condition in which a stimulus that is not painful in normal circumstances becomes painful). A state of hyperalgesia lasting at least 4 days has also been described in cows with mild or moderate mastitis. Kicking, irritability, and lack of milk flow when a cow's udder is gently manipulated during milking are signs of allodynia.

5.3.3 Prevention and husbandry recommendations

The most important risk factors identified in the report published by the European Food Safety Authority (EFSA 2009b, 2012) are **poor bedding hygiene** (especially for environmental pathogens) and poorly designed, managed, or maintained **milking equipment** (especially for contagious pathogens). Poor bedding should not only be avoided for lactating cows but also for dry and periparturient cows. Contact of the udder with dirty surfaces will increase the risk of mastitis (Figure 5.4).

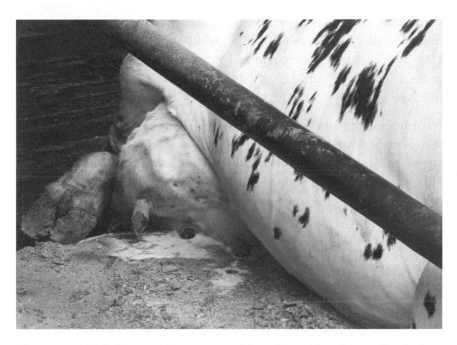

Figure 5.4 Milk leakage and/or contact of the udder with a dirty surface before or after milking increases the risk of mastitis.

The cows' environment, especially the lying and walking areas and the milking parlour, should be clean, dry and well ventilated. Milking equipment should be used and maintained to manufacturers' specifications to avoid trauma to the teats and udder. Infection prevention and control protocols should be carefully implemented during the milking routine (e.g. adequate teat preparation and disinfection, milking healthy cows first and infected cows afterwards). Robotic milking systems should be carefully adjusted and checked every day.

Early identification, monitoring, and treatment of mastitis in both the lactation and dry periods are extremely important. Similarly, the incidence of mastitis should be reduced by culling persistently infected cows and by improving the cows' immune system, by minimizing the stress factors to which they are exposed and by the provision of controlled amounts of a nutritionally balanced feed. Cows with severe mastitis and systemic signs of disease should be housed in a separate area; for these cows, adequate nutrition and a non-stressful environment are especially important to help ensure proper functioning of the immune system.

Pain management should be part of the treatment of clinical mastitis. A treatment protocol including antibiotics and anti-inflammatory drugs is recommended in cases of clinical mastitis. The efficacy of NSAIDs in alleviating the clinical signs associated with mastitis is greater than that of glucocorticoids, and for this reason NSAIDs can be considered as the drugs of choice for treating the pain and inflammation associated with mastitis. In studies of cows with experimentally induced mastitis, the use of NSAIDs decreases signs of udder inflammation and pain, maintains rumen motility, decreases rectal temperature and heart rate, and, in some studies, improves feed intake and milk yield. Although there have been few studies on the effect of NSAIDs on naturally occurring mastitis, a reduction of pain has been reported, and the use of NSAIDs has also been shown to reduce heart and respiratory rates, SCC, and the rate of culling. Overall, cows with mastitis recover faster when treated with NSAIDs compared with cows that receive only antibiotics.

Vaccine development against common udder pathogens has been advancing in the past few decades. The most targeted udder pathogens are *S. aureus*, *S. agalactiae*, and *E. coli*. Vaccination is one tool that could be used to prevent mastitis. However, vaccination alone is not necessarily effective or economical, especially in dairy herds with high rates of mastitis. Multiple factors account for the lack of success of vaccination, including inadequate vaccine targets, high diversity among mastitis-provoking strains of bacteria, cow-to-cow variation in the immune response, and failure to elicit an immune response that is appropriate for protection against a highly complex pathogen. The combination of vaccination and the application of other preventive and management measures described above usually results in a significant reduction in the incidence and duration of mastitis in a herd.

5.4 Painful husbandry practices: dehorning and disbudding

Dehorning and disbudding are relatively routine practices in cattle. This is mainly because polled animals are easier to handle and dehorning decreases the risk of injury to both people and other animals (Figure 5.5). Polled animals also require less space in the pen and at the feeder than horned animals. The most commonly used procedures are **hot-iron disbudding**, **chemical disbudding** (through the application of a caustic paste), and amputation dehorning. Whereas disbudding is usually performed during the first weeks of the animal's life (3–6 weeks), when the horn buds are between 5 mm and 10 mm long, dehorning is performed once the horn is formed.

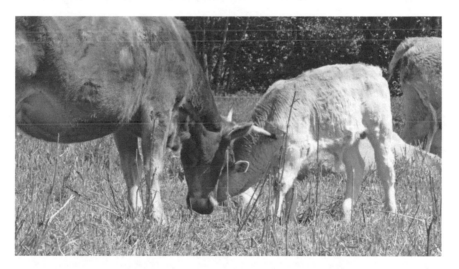

Figure 5.5 Horns increase the risk of injuries among herdmates.

'Dehorning is the term that may be applied to horn removal in cattle of all ages, while disbudding refers to removal of the horn buds in calves up to around 2 months of age.'

5.4.1 Dehorning and disbudding are painful practices

Although disbudding is justified for handling reasons and even on animal welfare grounds, it is nevertheless undeniably painful practice. The main behavioural, physiological, and production indicators of pain caused by dehorning and disbudding are shown in Table 5.7. In addition to acute pain, injuries due to disbudding can cause prolonged inflammation that can persist until the wound is healed, which can take months in some cases.

Although newborn animals have traditionally been thought to be less sensitive to pain than adults, this does not seem to be the case. In fact, animals of the so-called precocial species (i.e. those born in highly advanced stages of motor and sensory development), such as cattle, can experience pain even before birth. Even if the capacity to experience

Table 5.7 Behavioural, physiological, and production indicators of pain caused by dehorning and disbudding.

Behavioural indicators	Physiological and production indicators
Increased	Increased
Standing/lying events	Plasma cortisol
Tail shaking	Salivary cortisol
Head shaking	Heart rate
Head rubbing	Respiratory rate
Ear flicking	
Kicking	
Scratching	
Decreased	Decreased
Feeding and ruminating	Weight gain
Play behaviour	

pain increases gradually, the evidence seems to suggest that ruminants are already highly sensitive to pain at only a few hours after birth. In addition, some authors (Casoni et al., 2019; Adcock and Tucker, 2020) suggest that painful experiences in neonates can alter the development of neural pain pathways, leading to a systemic increase in pain sensitivity that can persist into adulthood.

Hot-iron disbudding

Hot-iron disbudding causes pain-related behavioural changes both during and after the procedure. These changes last about 4 h. Hot-iron disbudding damages the skin around the horn buds, leaving a relatively shallow wound. Hot-iron disbudding causes a slight increase in the total plasma cortisol concentration, which peaks at 30 min and returns to pre-treatment levels 2–4 h later.

Chemical disbudding

With chemical disbudding, the calf does not usually show signs of pain during the procedure. However, pain-related behavioural changes are observed after the procedure and can last up to 3–4 h. Moreover, the caustic paste that is applied can cause deep wounds in the treated animal and even in other animals because of physical contact between animals. Chemical disbudding causes a rise in plasma cortisol concentrations within 1 h of application of the caustic paste, and the cortisol concentration returns to pre-treatment levels 4–24 h later.

Amputation dehorning

Amputation dehorning causes behavioural changes during the procedure and for 6–8 h afterwards. Amputation affects the skin, bone, and sometimes the frontal sinus, causing deeper and more extensive lesions. Dehorning causes an immediate increase in plasma cortisol concentrations, which peak after about 30 min and return to pre-treatment levels 5–9 h later.

5.4.2 Minimizing or managing pain when disbudding

Dehorning should not be performed as it is extremely painful. Hot-iron disbudding is preferable to chemical disbudding or dehorning. Based on physiological and behavioural responses, hot-iron disbudding seems to be less painful than chemical disbudding.

Whenever possible, a combination of local anaesthesia and systemic analgesia using a NSAID should be used. Local anaesthesia is achieved by desensitization of the cornual nerve with an anaesthetic agent (Table 5.8). The local anaesthetic is injected just ventrally to the lateral edge of the frontal bone, midway from the base of the horn to the lateral canthus of the eye. Desensitization of the cornual tissue should be confirmed by assessing the animal's behavioural reactions (e.g. ear flicking or strong escape behaviour) to a needle prick several minutes after administration of the cornual nerve block. If a response is observed to this needle prick, administration of an anaesthetic agent should be repeated in the same manner as described above. Following confirmation of appropriate desensitization, calves are cautery disbudded by the placement of a preheated hot-iron on the horn tissue for approximately 10 s.

Table 5.8 Options for local anaesthesia and systemic analgesia that have been shown to mitigate pain associated with hot-iron disbudding (based on Winder et al., 2018).

Local anaesthesia (cornual nerve block)		
Active substance	Dose (each site)	Time of administration
Lidocaine 2%	5 ml	5–15 min before disbudding
Lidocaine HCl 2% with adrenaline (epinephrine)	5–6 ml	10–20 min before disbudding
Lignocaine HCl 2%	3–5 ml	10–20 min before disbudding
Procaine HCl 2%	10 ml	20 min before disbudding

Non-steroidal anti-inflammatory drug (systemic analgesia)			
Active substance	Route	Dose	Time of administration
Carprofen	O	1.4 mg/kg	10 min before disbudding
		2.0 mg/kg	5 min before disbudding
	SC	1.4 mg/kg	10 min before disbudding
	IV	1.4 mg/kg	15 min before disbudding
Dexketoprofen	IV	3.0 mg/kg	30 min before disbudding
Firocoxib	O	0.5 mg/kg	10 min before disbudding
		2.0 mg/kg	5 min before disbudding
Flunixin meglumine	O	2.3 mg/kg	5 min before disbudding
	IV	2.2 mg/kg	At disbudding and 3 h after disbudding
Ketoprofen	O	3.0 mg/kg	12 h before disbudding, and 2 h and 7 h after disbudding
	IM	3.0 mg/kg	10 min pre-disbud
Meloxicam	O	1.0 mg/kg	At disbudding or 12 h before disbudding
		2.0 mg/kg	5 min before disbudding
	IM	0.5 mg/kg	10 min before disbudding
	IV	0.5 mg/kg	55 min before disbudding

Route: O = oral; SC = subcutaneous; IV = intravenous; IM = intramuscular.

The use of local anaesthesia and post-operative analgesia in this way will virtually eliminate all behavioural and hormonal changes indicative of acute pain caused by disbudding. As calves may experience chronic pain for 24–48 h after disbudding, extending the analgesic treatment to cover this period should be considered.

Sedation (e.g. with xylazine) has been studied alone and in combination with local anaesthesia. The combination decreases the cortisol response and the physical activity of calves during disbudding, but sedation alone does not eliminate the peak cortisol response and has a limited effect on head movements during disbudding. Thus, the use of sedation with xylazine without anaesthesia is not recommended, as xylazine alone does not control the pain associated with disbudding.

European recommendations

The current European legislation regarding minimum standards for the protection of calves (Directive 91/629/ECC) does not regulate dehorning or disbudding procedures. Nevertheless, in some countries it is now mandatory to provide pain relief during painful procedures. Moreover, according to the UK Code of Recommendations for the Welfare of Cattle, disbudding should be performed before calves are 2 months old and, ideally, as soon as the horn bud is visible. It is strongly recommended that chemical disbudding should not be used, and hot-iron disbudding should be carried out under local anaesthesia by a trained and competent stockperson. Dehorning should not be a routine procedure, and the use of polled cattle breeds must be considered as an alternative to dehorning in the future.

Bibliography

Adcock, S.J.J. and Tucker, C.B. (2018) The effect of disbudding age on healing and pain sensitivity in dairy calves. *Journal of Dairy Science* 101, 10361–10373.

Adcock, S.J.J. and Tucker, C.B. (2020) The effect of early burn injury on sensitivity to future painful stimuli in dairy heifers. *PLoS ONE* 15, e0233711.

Alsaaod, M., Fadul, M. and Steiner, A. (2019) Review: Automatic lameness detection in cattle. *The Veterinary Journal* 246, 35–44.

Anil, L., Anil, S.S. and Deen, J. (2005) Pain detection and amelioration in animals on the farm: issues and options. *Journal of Applied Animal Welfare Science* 8, 261–278.

Caray, D., Boyer des Roches, A., Frouja, S., Andanson, S. and Veissier, I. (2015) Hot-iron disbudding: stress responses and behavior of 1- and 4-week-old calves receiving anti-inflammatory analgesia without or with sedation using xylazine. *Livestock Science* 179, 22–28.

Casoni, D., Mirra, A., Suter, M.R., Gutzwiller, A. and Spadavecchia, C. (2019) Can disbudding of calves (one versus four weeks of age) induce chronic pain? *Physiology & Behavior* 199, 47–55.

Coetzee, J.F., Shearer, J.K., Stock, M.L., Kleinhenz, M.D. and van Amstel, S.R. (2017) An update on the assessment and management of pain associated with lameness in cattle. *Veterinary Clinics of North America: Food Animal Practice* 33, 389–411.

Cook, N.B. (2017) A review of the design and management of footbaths for dairy cattle. *Veterinary Clinics of North America: Food Animal Practice* 33, 195–225.

Côté-Gravel, J. and Malouin, F. (2019) Symposium review: Features of *Staphylococcus aureus* mastitis pathogenesis that guide vaccine development strategies. *Journal of Dairy Science* 102, 4727–4740.

Council of the European Union (1991) Council Directive 91/629/EEC of 19 November 1991 laying down minimum standards for the protection of calves. *Official Journal of the European Communities* L340, 28–32.

DEFRA (2003) Code of Recommendations for the Welfare of Livestock: Cattle. Available at: https://assets.publishing.service.gov.uk/government/uploads/system/uploads/attachment_data/file/69368/pb7949-cattle-code-030407.pdf (accessed 16 November 2021).

Dittrich, I., Gertz, M. and Krieter, J. (2019) Alterations in sick dairy cows' daily behavioural patterns. *Heliyon* 5, e02902.

EFSA (2009a) Scientific opinion on welfare of dairy cows in relation to leg and locomotion problems based on a risk assessment with special reference to the impact of housing, feeding, management and genetic selection. Scientific opinion of the Panel on Animal Health and Animal Welfare. *The EFSA Journal* 1142, 1–57.

EFSA (2009b) Scientific opinion on welfare of dairy cows in relation to udder problems based on a risk assessment with special reference to the impact of housing, feeding, management and genetic selection. Scientific opinion of the Panel on Animal Health and Animal Welfare. *The EFSA Journal* 1141, 1–60.

EFSA (2012) Scientific opinion on the use of animal-based measures to assess the welfare of dairy cows. EFSA Panel on Animal Health and Welfare. *The EFSA Journal* 10, 2554.

Gleerup, K.B., Andersen, P.H., Munksgaard, L. and Forkman, B. (2015) Pain evaluation in dairy cattle. *Applied Animal Behaviour Science* 171, 25–32.

Herskin, M.S. and Nielsen, B.H. (2018) Welfare effects of the use of a combination of local anesthesia and NSAID for disbudding analgesia in dairy calves—reviewed across different welfare concerns. *Frontiers in Veterinary Science* 5, 117.

Hogeveen, H., Huijps, K. and Lam, T.J.G.M. (2011) Economic aspects of mastitis: new developments. *New Zealand Veterinary Journal* 59, 16–23.

Ismail, Z.B. (2017) Mastitis vaccines in dairy cows: recent developments and recommendations of application. *Veterinary World* 10, 1057–1062.

Leslie, K.E. and Petersson-Wolfe, C.S. (2012) Assessment and management of pain in dairy cows with clinical mastitis. *Veterinary Clinics of North America: Food Animal Practice* 28, 289–305.

Mellor, D.J. and Diesch, T.J. (2006) Onset of sentience: the potential for suffering in fetal and newborn farm animals. *Applied Animal Behaviour Science* 100, 48–57.

Mirra, A., Spadavecchia, C., Bruckmaier, R., Gutzwiller, A. and Casoni, D. (2018) Acute pain and peripheral sensitization following disbudding in 1- and 4-week-old calves. *Physiology & Behavior* 184, 248–260.

O'Driscoll, K. (2016) Lameness. In: *Teagasc Dairy Manual.* Agriculture and Food Development Authority, Teagasc, Carlow, Ireland, pp. 295–298.

Polsky, L. and von Keyserlingk, M.A.G. (2017) Invited review: Effects of heat stress on dairy cattle welfare. *Journal of Dairy Science* 100, 8645–8657.

Rutten, C.J., Velthuis, A.G.J., Steeneveld, W. and Hogeveen, H. (2013) Invited review: Sensors to support health management on dairy farms. *Journal of Dairy Science* 96, 1928–1952.

Sadiq, M.B., Ramanoon, S.Z., Mossadeq, W.M.S., Mansor, R. and Syed-Hussain, S.S.S. (2017) Review: Association between lameness and indicators of dairy cow welfare based on locomotion scoring, body and hock condition, leg hygiene and lying behavior. *Animals* 7, 79–96.

Siivonen, J., Taponen, S., Hovinen, M., Pastell, M., Lensink, B.J., Pyörälä, S. and Hänninen, L. (2011) Impact of acute clinical mastitis on cow behaviour. *Applied Animal Behaviour Science* 132, 101–106.

Sprecher, D.J., Hostetler, D.E. and Kaneene, J.B. (1997) A lameness scoring system uses posture and gait to predict dairy cattle reproductive performance. *Theriogenology* 47, 1179–1187.

Stafford, K.J. and Mellor, D.J. (2011) Addressing the pain associated with disbudding and dehorning in cattle. *Applied Animal Behaviour Science* 135, 226–231.

Stock, M.L., Baldridge, S.L., Griffin, D. and Coetzee, J.F. (2013) Bovine dehorning. Assessing pain and providing analgesic management. *Veterinary Clinics of North America: Food Animal Practice* 29, 103–133.

Tadich, N., Tejeda, C., Bastias, S., Rosenfeld, C. and Green, L.E. (2013) Nociceptive threshold, blood constituents and physiological values in 213 cows with locomotion scores ranging from normal to severely lame. *The Veterinary Journal* 197, 401–405.

Vickers, K.J., Niel, L., Kiehlbauch, L.M. and Weary, D.M. (2005) Calf response to caustic paste and hot-iron dehorning using sedation with and without local anesthetic. *Journal of Dairy Science* 88, 1454–1459.

Weigele, H.C., Gygax, L., Steiner, A., Wechsler, B. and Burla, J.-B. (2018) Moderate lameness leads to marked behavioural changes in dairy cows. *Journal of Dairy Science* 101, 2370–2382.

Whay, H.R. (2002) Locomotion scoring and lameness detection in dairy cattle. *In Practice* 24, 444–449.

Whay, H.R. and Shearer, J.K. (2017) The impact of lameness on welfare of the dairy cow. *Veterinary Clinics of North America: Food Animal Practice* 33, 153–164.

Winder, C.B., Miltenburg, C.L., Sargeant, J.M., LeBlanc, S.J., Haley, D.B., Lissemore, K.D., Godkin, M.A. and Duffield, T.F. (2018) Effects of local anesthetic or systemic analgesia on pain associated with cautery disbudding in calves: a systematic review and meta-analysis. *Journal of Dairy Science* 101, 5411–5427.

CHAPTER 6

Welfare issues related to behaviour

During domestication, farm animal species have been bred to increase their productivity and have undergone changes in their physiology and anatomy. Although their behaviour has changed as an adaptation to farming conditions, their behavioural needs remain intact. Therefore, they show a strong preference to perform their natural behaviours, and expression of these behaviours is key to safeguarding animal welfare. Behaviour is also very important as it can help to identify animal welfare problems.

6.1 Mixing animals and hierarchy

The expression of **social behaviour** is one of the most important natural behaviours of farm animals. Social behaviour can be classified as positive or negative. Positive social behaviour will be beneficial for the welfare of animals whereas negative behaviour will be harmful and result in the animals experiencing stress, anxiety, or frustration. Therefore, positive social behaviour should be prioritized as opposed to negative behaviour. Examples of positive social behaviours are allogrooming or social licking (Figure 6.1) and mutually touching horns (or heads in dehorned cattle). Inter-individual bonds and preferential relationships are mainly established, maintained, and reinforced through these positive social behaviours.

The ancestors of farm animals developed a social structure as a strategy to defend against predators. It is assumed that if animals live in groups,

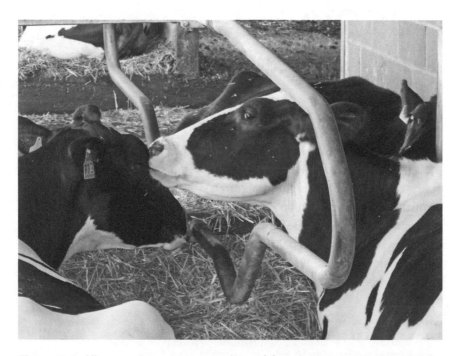

Figure 6.1 Allogrooming serves a variety of functions in cattle. Besides its hygienic function and the provision of pleasure, it is also known to serve several social purposes. Allogrooming enhances group cohesion and maintains social stability, reduces social tension, and has calming effects.

since they are gregarious, every individual animal will have a smaller chance of being caught by any predator. This strategy needs animals to communicate with each other, for example, to alert others in the group about the presence of predators, but it also implies that competition will exist if resources are limited. For example, if a large group of animals settles in an area with a small supply of food, it will not be able to feed all individuals of the group, and so competition for food will arise.

Hierarchy is used in gregarious species to establish the order for accessing resources. This strategy means that the stronger animals, which are possibly more fit for reproduction, will have access to resources first, thus facilitating continuation of the species.

> *'Hierarchy is the social structure of gregarious species used to establish the order for having access to resources.'*

Groups of animals establish a hierarchy through negative social behaviours such as aggression. For example, if in any group of animals resources such as food or space are limited, the stronger or fitter animals will use aggressive behaviour to displace other animals, thus guaranteeing their access to the limited resource. If the displacement is successful, the aggressor will become the dominant animal and the aggressed will be the subordinate. Although the most recurrent form of aggressive behaviour is fighting, there are many other forms that do not necessarily imply physical harm. For example, cattle use chasing, pushing, or head butting to threaten other animals.

6.2 Competition for resources

Any resource can be a source of competition and conflict when it is limited. As well as food or water, as mentioned, other limited resources, such as comfortable resting places or ventilated areas, can lead to competition. When resources are scarce, animals use aggressive behaviour to access them according to the hierarchy. More dominant and aggressive animals will access food before the subordinate animals. Dominant animals may abuse their position in the hierarchy and deny the subordinate animals sufficient access to food, resulting in not only malnutrition but also frustration and stress.

Although cattle do not often engage in severe aggression during competition for food, it can sometimes result in distress and minor injuries (e.g. skin lesions). Dominant cows hoard the feeding place and displace subordinate cows. As an example, a supposedly dominant cow might try to displace another cow from the feeding area by head butting. The pressure put on the subordinate cow to displace her will decrease her feed intake. To avoid excessive competition in the feeding area, it is recommended that there be 10% more feeding spaces (if they are individual headlocks) than the number of cows in the pen. For example, a pen containing 70 cows should have 77 effective individual feeding spaces.

> 'There should be 10% more individual feeding spaces than the current number of cows in the pen.'

In situations where feeding spaces are not individual, the recommendation to prevent feeding competition is to provide no less than 60 cm space per adult cow. If this minimum space is not provided, the average feed intake of the herd will decrease. For instance, in feeding areas that have less than 20 cm per cow present in the pen, there is a significant reduction of both feed intake and feeding time.

Divisions at the feeder separating the heads of individuals that are side by side allow subordinate cows better access to the feed. In fact, evidence suggests that cows with lower feeding times relative to their groupmates when accessing a feeder with a post-and-rail barrier showed more similar feeding times to their groupmates when using a feeder with a headlock barrier.

In cattle, rapid ingestion of feed is associated with rapid rumen fermentation and a greater risk of acidosis. This is particularly the case if the feed contains a high proportion of concentrates. Increasing the feeding space has positive effects on both feed intake (cows eat more feed) and feeding time (cows eat more slowly), which increases productivity and reduces the risk of acidosis, respectively.

In addition to the length of the feeding space, designs that allow individualization of the feeding space can reduce competition at the feeder. A useful study reveals the impact of separation of the feeder into individual spaces using different designs to separate the individual feeding spaces (Bouissou, 1980). In the study, two dairy cows were introduced to an experimental pen with food in a single feeding trough, and were left for 3 min. In the first situation, the subordinate cow was able to access the food only for 7 s, whereas the dominant cow spent almost all the time eating. Although the best situation in terms of equality in feeding time occurred where there is a complete separation between the two feeding spaces, it is worth noting that a slight separation between spaces can have a very similar result in reducing competition for feed.

6.3 Fear and the human–animal relationship

The quality of stockpersons has an important effect on the welfare and performance of dairy cattle. Indeed, the attitude of the stockpersons when interacting with their animals mostly determines whether cattle are more or less fearful of people. Fear affects milk production and has pronounced negative effects on animal welfare. Positive interactions with the cows, by contrast, can also positively improve their health status. To prevent fearfulness, a positive human–animal relationship should be fostered as early as possible in the life of the animal.

6.3.1 What is fear?

Fear is defined as an unpleasant emotional experience caused by a stimulus that the animal perceives as a threat. In general, two kinds of stimuli can cause fear. First, **intense sensory stimuli**, such as a sudden noise, trigger a fear response without involving a learning process. Second, animals may learn to associate a **neutral stimulus**, such as the presence of humans, with a **negative experience**, such as being slapped, shouted at or pushed, due to a conditioning learning process. Moreover, according to some authors (see Waiblinger et al., 2006 for further review), domesticated animals may perceive humans as predators and, to a certain extent, are thus 'predisposed' to associate the presence of humans with negative stimuli. Fear is also affected by the genetic make-up of the animals, and has shown a medium-to-high heritability.

Pheromones play an important role in communication between cows, and one pheromone that is particularly relevant here is the so-called alarm pheromone. In a frightening situation, cows secrete a volatile molecule or set of molecules (which are synthesized in the cutaneous glands located between the hooves) that induce fear and stress in other cows. So, a situation that causes fear in one cow may affect the entire herd.

Fear triggers a set of behavioural – mainly, the flight response – and physiological changes. In general, the physiological changes associated with fear are similar to the stress response and have negative effects on feed intake, rumination, milk production, and fertility. The fear response inhibits the synthesis and release of oxytocin, which is responsible for the milk ejection reflex, and this largely explains the importance of human–animal interactions in the milking parlour.

'Positive interactions with the cows may reduce fear towards humans, therefore improving their welfare and milk production.'

6.3.2 Prevention of fear through good human–cow interactions

The **quality of stockpersons** and their relationship with the cows has a strong impact on their everyday work. Fearful animals are much more difficult to handle; for example, they are unpredictable and may react suddenly. This represents a major risk to personnel. In fact, most accidents on dairy cow farms are due to the reaction of fearful animals. Positive human–animal interactions not only facilitate animal handling but also contribute to better job satisfaction for the stockperson.

Cows perceive interactions with humans as either aversive, positive, or neutral, depending on the quality of the interaction. Dairy cows experience a number of handling procedures throughout their lives, such as oestrus detection and subsequent artificial insemination, potential interventions to assist parturition, movement from one place to another, vaccinations and other necessary treatments that can be painful. These situations can easily be perceived by the cow as aversive. Good management can significantly decrease the fear response of the animal, even when experiencing some procedures that are painful but necessary. Positive handling of the cows for a short period of time daily can successfully reduce their fearfulness, triggering direct benefits in their productive and reproductive performance.

Studies published in dairy cows indicate that the most important parameter that determines the cows' fear of humans is the proportion of negative interactions out of the total number of interactions between the farmer and the animals. Cows that are regularly handled in a positive way usually show less fear of humans than those that have reduced contact with humans. Regular positive handling results not only in less agitated behaviour when cows are in close proximity to humans but also in a lower heart rate and a lower plasma cortisol concentration, which are indicative of a reduced stress response.

The most frequent negative interactions involve the cows being pushed and hit by the stockperson when they are being moved, especially to the milking parlour. By contrast, positive interactions include the stock-person patting or touching the cows gently and resting their hand on the back of the cows during milking. The stockperson's voice is also an important signal that can be used in daily activities such as milking, feeding, or cleaning. Speaking to the cows with a calm tone of voice will facilitate the establishment of a positive interaction with the cows, whereas shouting will alarm them.

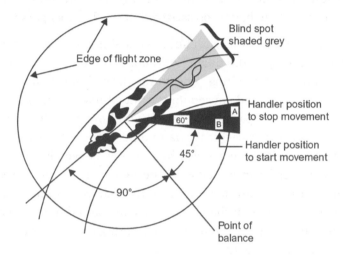

Flight zone = area that if encroached upon by humans causes escape behaviour.

- **Position A** = outside the flight zone.
- **Position B** = inside the flight zone.
- **When moving from position A to B**, the handler exerts a 'pressure' on the animal to move.

Point of balance = the animal will move forwards if the handler walks behind this point and backwards if the handler walks beyond this point.

Blind spot = area where the animal cannot see the handler.

Figure 6.2 Recommended handler position for driving cattle (reprinted from *Genetics and the Behavior of Domestic Animals*, Temple Grandin, Mark J. Deesing, Copyright (2014), with permission from Elsevier).

Cows and stockpersons interact most frequently during milking and when the cows are being moved to and from the milking parlour. Moving the animals can be stressful, especially if it is done in an inappropriate way or if the facilities are not adequate. Figure 6.2 shows the recommended position of the handler to drive cows in a gentle way.

6.3.3 Assessment of fear towards humans

A cow's fear of people triggers a series of behaviour changes that can be measured by several indicators such as the so-called 'flight distance', the latency time in the approach of the animal to the observer, or the time during which the animal will stay still close to the observer.

The way in which cows react to humans is included in several welfare evaluation systems, such as the 'human–animal relationship' test from the Welfare Quality® protocol. This test evaluates the human–animal relationship by the flight distance, measured individually. The person doing the test should initially be about 2 m away from the head of the cow in the area of the feeders and move slowly towards the cow with their arm held in front of them forming a 45° angle with the ground and the palm of their hand downwards (Figure 6.3). The person should not look directly into the eyes of the cow. The distance between the tip of the fingers of the hand and the cow's muzzle when the cow makes the first movement of flight (i.e. moving away from the person) should be recorded. Thus, two types of measurements are obtained: the percentage of cows that allow themselves to be touched and the average flight distance. The human–animal relationship is considered good when the average flight distance is less than 50 cm and most cows allow themselves to be touched by the person.

Welfare assessment protocols usually evaluate the fear of strangers, since the observations are made by an assessor who does not habitually interact with the animals.

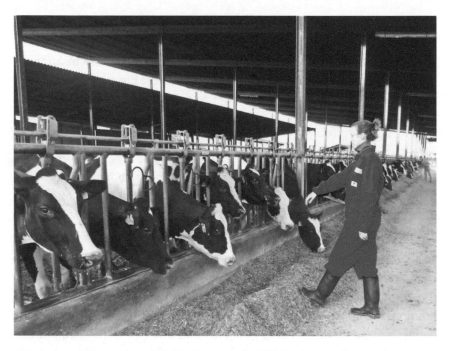

Figure 6.3 Assessor conducting the so-called 'flight distance' test, which measures the quality of the human–animal relationship.

Bibliography

Boissy, A. (1995) Fear and fearfulness in animals. *Quarterly Review of Biology* 70, 165–191.

Bouissou, M.-F. (1980) Social relationships in domestic cattle under modern management techniques. *Italian Journal of Zoology* 47, 343–353.

de Passillé, A.M. and Rushen, J. (2005) Can we measure human–animal interactions in on-farm animal welfare assessment? Some unresolved issues. *Applied Animal Behaviour Science* 92, 193–209.

Endres, M.I., DeVries, T.J., von Keyserlingk, M.A.G. and Weary, D.M. (2005) Effect of feed barrier design on the behavior of loose-housed lactating dairy cows. *Journal of Dairy Science 88*, 2377–2380.

Fallahi, S. (2019) Behavioral genetics in cattle – a review. *Journal of Livestock Science* 10, 102–108.

Fregonesi, J.A., Tucker, C.B. and Weary, D.M. (2007) Overstocking reduces lying time in dairy cows. *Journal of Dairy Science* 90, 3349–3354.

González, L.A., Manteca, X., Calsamiglia, S., Schwartzkopf-Genswein, K.S. and Ferret, A. (2012) Ruminal acidosis in feedlot cattle: interplay between feed ingredients, rumen function and feeding behavior (a review). *Animal Feed Science and Technology* 172, 66–79.

Grandin, T. (1980) Observations of cattle behaviour applied to the design of cattle handling facilities. *Applied Animal Ethology* 6, 19–31.

Grandin, T. and Deesing, M.J. (2014) *Genetics and the Behavior of Domestic Animals*, 2nd edn. Academic Press, Cambridge, MA.

Hemsworth, P.H., Coleman, G.J., Barnett, J.L. and Borg, S. (2000) Relationships between human-animal interactions and productivity of commercial dairy cows. *Journal of Animal Science* 78, 2821–2831.

Jones, R.B. and Boissy, A. (2011) Fear and other negative emotions. In: Appleby, M.C., Mench, J.A., Olsson, I.A.S. and Hughes, B.O. (eds) *Animal Welfare*, 2nd edn. CAB International, Wallingford, UK, pp. 78–97.

Keeling, J.L. and Gonyou, H.W. (2001) *Social Behavior in Farm Animals*, 1st edn. CABI Publishing, Wallingford, UK.

Mota-Rojas, D., Broom, D.M., Orihucla, A., Velarde, A., Napolitano F. and Alonso-Spilsbury, M. (2020) Effects of human-animal relationship on animal productivity and welfare. *Journal of Animal Behaviour and Biometeorology* 8, 196–205.

Pajor, E.A., Rushen, J. and de Passillé, A.M. (2000) Aversion learning techniques to evaluate dairy cattle handling practices. *Applied Animal Behaviour Science* 69, 89–102.

Proudfoot, K.L., Veira, D.M., Weary, D.M. and von Keyserlingk, M.A.G. (2009) Competition at the feed bunk changes the feeding, standing, and social behavior of transition dairy cows. *Journal of Dairy Science* 92, 3116–3123.

Rousing, T. and Waiblinger, S. (2004) Evaluation of on-farm methods for testing the human–animal relationship in dairy herds with cubicle loose housing systems: test–retest and inter-observer reliability and consistency to familiarity of test person. *Applied Animal Behaviour Science* 85, 215–231.

Val-Laillet, D., Guesdon, V., von Keyserlingk, M.A.G. and Rushen, J. (2009) Allogrooming in cattle: relationships between social preferences, feeding displacements and social dominance. *Applied Animal Behaviour Science* 116, 141–149.

Waiblinger, S., Boivin, X., Perdersen, V., Tosi, M.V., Janczak, A.M., Visser, E.K. and Jones, R.B. (2006) Assessing the human–animal relationship in farmed species: a critical review. *Applied Animal Behaviour Science* 101, 185–242.

Waiblinger, S., Menke, C. and Fölsch, D.W. (2003) Influences on the avoidance and approach behaviour of dairy cows towards humans on 35 farms. *Applied Animal Behaviour Science* 84, 23–39.

CHAPTER 7

Welfare at milking

Milking is considered one of the most important routine tasks performed by dairy cattle farmers and is also rated as the most enjoyable task. Milking is also the most frequent direct interaction between dairy cows and the stockperson. Chronic pain associated with diseases or injuries and any stressful situations occurring during milking are likely to result in a decrease in milk yield.

7.1 Health problems related to milking

In terms of diseases and injuries directly related to milking, special attention should be given to the prevention of teat injuries and mastitis (especially when contagious mastitis microorganisms are involved). Mastitis is more likely to develop at the time of peak milk yield, and cows with a high milk flow rate may be more prone to pick up infections through the teat canal. Some evidence suggests that the incidence of mastitis may be reduced by increasing the frequency of milking. On the other hand, increasing the frequency of milking may also increase the risk of teat damage and secondary invasion by environmental pathogens after each milking.

'Routine tasks of animal care, such as teat disinfection and cleaning, and the management of the milking equipment are of major importance in ensuring good animal health during milking.'

Pain is a stress factor that must not be forgotten. Poor practices in the milking parlour can cause pain. In addition, chronic pain (e.g. that associated with lameness or mastitis) will inevitably result in the inhibition of milk ejection. Therefore, pain must be prevented wherever possible, and treated when painful conditions do arise.

The practice of over-milking produces an increase in the behavioural indicators of pain. This is because the cow feels discomfort in the udder resulting from the prolonged and greater exposure of the teats to a vacuum. Therefore, it is recommended that the liners (or teat cup liners) be removed immediately after the milk flow has stopped.

Lameness or mastitis cause chronic pain, which has a negative effect on the cows' welfare and yield. In the case of lameness, it is recommended to open accommodation areas for lame cows near the milking parlour to reduce the distance these animals must walk each day. Some behaviours indicating lameness may be apparent while the cows are standing in the milking parlour; for example, arching of the back, the so-called 'cow-hocked' stance (see section 5.2.3), or when the animal supports its weight on one limb because the contralateral limb is painful. In cases of lameness and clinical mastitis, treatment with a non-steroidal anti-inflammatory drug (NSAID) is recommended to relieve the pain (see also sections 5.2 and 5.3).

Note on automatic milking

Automatic milking is an increasingly common practice in dairy production. With respect to the welfare of the cow, the use of automatic milking systems has both advantages and disadvantages, and some recent studies conclude that automatic milking and conventional milking are equally acceptable in terms of dairy-cow welfare (Table 7.1).

Table 7.1 Main advantages and disadvantages of automatic milking in relation to the welfare of the cows.

Advantages	Disadvantages
Increase in milking frequency and possible improvement of udder health	Higher risk of poor positioning of the teat cup liners, causing drips and an increased risk of mastitis
Cows visit the milking unit whenever they want to. This gives them more control over their environment	Subordinate animals may be forced to go to the milking machine at night

7.2 Indicators of stress during milking

Acute stress during milking reduces milk yield through a central inhibition of oxytocin secretion and the peripheral actions of catecholamines. Oxytocin, a hormone secreted by the central nervous system into the bloodstream, is the main mediator of the milk ejection reflex. The secretion of oxytocin is thus of major importance to optimize milk production. A variety of acute stressors, such as social isolation, novel surroundings (especially for heifers), pain associated with diseases or injuries, or fear of the people present at milking lead to the inhibition of milk ejection.

Besides its impact on productivity, the behavioural response of cows to a stressful situation also increases the risk of injury for the stockperson.

'30% of the variability in annual milk production among farms can be attributed to differences in the degree of fearfulness of the cows.'

Several behavioural indicators can be useful to identify welfare problems related to milking.

- **Stepping** during milking can be an indicator of general discomfort (e.g. chronic pain or over-milking) or fear of the personnel who are present. A higher frequency of stepping behaviour is observed in anxious and nervous animals. Cows that are managed gently show a shorter flight distance (the distance between a person approaching the animal and the animal itself at the moment of withdrawal; see section 6.3.3) and less stepping behaviour during milking.
- Cows that experience pain due to teat lesions are more likely to **kick** during milking. In contrast, fearful cows do not usually show kicking behaviour. Kicking is also an indicator of discomfort caused by low milk flow and vacuum milking.
- **Defecation, urination, and vocalization** in the milking parlour are indicators of acute stress and fear in cows (Figure 7.1). These behaviours increase when the cows are isolated or introduced into novel surroundings. Interestingly, the occurrence of these indicators decreases in the presence of the stockperson (when the

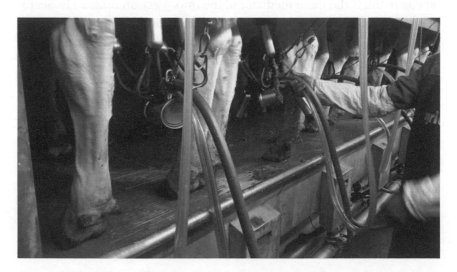

Figure 7.1 Defecation may be observed during the first milking of primiparous cows. Defecation is rarely observed in the subsequent milkings of primiparous cows and in multiparous cows, unless there is a problem of fear or stress at milking.

human–animal relationship is good). The presence of a person who has a good relationship with the cows may therefore reduce the fear responses of cows during milking.

7.3 Preventing stress during milking through good management routines

The presence of a handler who interacts with the cows in an aversive way (e.g. with sudden and unpredictable movements, shouting, and/or slapping) during milking is enough to cause the cows to 'hold back' milk due to the suppression of oxytocin secretion. Studies comparing farms with similar environmental conditions and cows with the same genetic background have shown that farms with the highest productivity are those with stockpersons who speak to and touch their cows more often. The animals are in turn less frightened, less reluctant to be driven, and more likely to approach the stockperson. Under controlled conditions, just the presence of an aversive handler during milking is enough to increase residual milk by 70%, and therefore reduce milk yield.

It is, then, important to take advantage of each milking event to optimize the interaction between the stockperson and the cows, and to avoid using some routine behaviours that could result in cows becoming fearful.

- Maximize positive contacts such as talking calmly, patting the cows, and moving slowly and in a predictable manner.
- Minimize negative contacts such as shouting at or slapping the cows, or making fast and unexpected movements.
- Providing small food rewards when dairy cows enter the milking parlour may reduce the time they take to enter the parlour, which in turn reduces the need to push the cows or use other aversive handling techniques.

Handling of cows during milking must be done with patience and sensitivity. The person in charge should be familiar with the behaviour of the cows and the best ways to manage them. Above all, this person must be aware of the importance of handling to help ensure the welfare of the cows at milking.

7.3.1 Moving the cows towards the waiting area

It is important to move the cows to the waiting area calmly, without running or shouting. Ideally, the cows will walk to the waiting area on their own. It is recommended that moving the animals should always be carried out by the same person, and at the same times of day. The animals can be stimulated to walk by talking to them, whistling, walking in a 'zigzag' pattern behind them and, when necessary, gently tapping their hind legs or back with the hand.

Cows are animals that like routines: they prefer to go along the same roads, lie down in the same place, and drink water at the same time and from the same drinker. These activities are usually carried out in groups, under the influence of one or several individuals, who are the 'leader' cows. Leadership is defined when an animal starts to move or chooses a certain place to do an activity (e.g. rest) and is followed by the other animals in the group. The leader cow is usually the oldest of the group, but this is not always the case. It is easier for the stockperson to move groups of cows to the milking parlour when they can identify the leader cow in each group. Stimulating the leader cow to move can encourage the other cows to follow her and accompany her into the waiting area.

7.3.2 In the milking parlour

When the cows are in the waiting area, it is recommended to wait a few minutes before starting the other activities, to give them time to recover. It is better not to place too many cows in the waiting area at the same time. The waiting area is usually not a comfortable space (e.g. it might have a high stocking density and/or be noisy), and this can cause the cows discomfort and stress. In addition, having small groups in the waiting area facilitates their management and entry to the milking parlour.

It is advisable not to force the cows into the milking parlour and to respect their preferred order to access the parlour. It is important to remember that the so-called 'waiting room pusher' should be used only to delimit the waiting area, and in no case to push the cows. The presence of electric shocks (even at low intensity) should be eliminated completely in the milking parlour. Likewise, it is recommended to respect the preferences of each animal when choosing their milking place.

To reduce stress during milking, it is important that cows can anticipate each task in the milking parlour. Giving signals to the animals is very useful to help them anticipate each procedure and minimize the risk that they will react with fear. For example, it is advisable to touch the udder before placing the teat cup liners.

Good management of cows during milking is essential to maximize their milk production. However, we must not forget that the people in charge of milking also have other fundamental responsibilities, such as compliance with milking schedules, cleaning and preparation of the room, and detecting animals with possible health problems.

Positive management of cows pays off

In a study in Canada by Rushen et al. (1999) dairy cows were repeatedly handled by two persons, one of whom always handled the cows in a smooth and gentle manner (speaking in a low voice, stroking the cows, and occasionally giving rewards of food) whereas the other handled the cows in an aversive manner (shouting, being abrupt, and occasionally using a plastic shovel to strike the cows).

The cows' fear of each of these two people was evaluated by means of an approach test in the feeding area. The results showed that after several

continued

repetitions of the 'fear tests', the cows remained further away from the 'aversive' operator than from the 'gentle' operator. The authors of the study evaluated whether the degree of fear caused by the type of management was enough to reduce milk production. They milked the cows in the presence of each of the two workers. The mere presence of the aversive operator during milking was enough to increase residual milk by 70% (which indicates a blockage of milk ejection induced by the stress response) and significantly reduce milk production. Some physiological changes were also detected: in the presence of the aversive operator, the cows had a higher heart rate during milking.

Training of stockpersons improves cow welfare and productivity

A study conducted in Australia by Hemsworth et al. (2002) evaluated the effect of a special training programme to improve farmers' attitudes towards the dairy cows they manage. Of the 141 stockpersons who were present, half participated in the training programme while the other half remained as a control group. The stockpersons who participated in the training programme changed their way of managing cows, and began using less aversive signals and more positive interactions with the animals. In addition, the escape distance of the cows in front of a person was smaller on the farms where the stockpersons had followed the training programme. Finally, improvements in cow management had a positive impact on productive yields.

Bibliography

Breuer, K., Hemsworth, P.H., Barnett, J.L., Matthews, L.R. and Coleman, G.J. (2000) Behavioural response to humans and the productivity of commercial dairy cows. *Applied Animal Behaviour Science* 66, 273–288.

Hemsworth, P.H., Barnett, J.L., Tilbrook, A.J. and Hansen, C. (1989) The effects of handling by humans at calving and during milking on the behaviour and milk cortisol concentrations of primiparous dairy cows. *Applied Animal Behaviour Science* 22, 313–326.

Hemsworth, P.H. and Coleman, G.J. (2010) The stockperson and the productivity and welfare of intensively farmed animals. In: Hemsworth, P.H. and Coleman, G.H. (eds) *Human–Livestock Interactions,* 2nd edn. CABI international, Wallingford, UK, pp. 47–87.

Hemsworth, P.H., Coleman, G.J., Barnett, J.L. and Borg, S. (2000) Relationships between human-animal interactions and productivity of commercial dairy cows. *Journal of Animal Science* 78, 2821–2831.

Hemsworth, P.H., Coleman, G.J., Barnett, J.L., Borg, S., and Dowling, S. (2002) The effects of cognitive behavioral intervention on the attitude and behavior of stockpersons and the behavior and productivity of commercial dairy cows. *Journal of Animal Science* 80, 68–78.

Hogeveen, H., Huijps, K. and Lam, T.J.G.M. (2011) Economic aspects of mastitis: new developments. *New Zealand Veterinary Journal 59, 16–23.*

Hopster, H., Bruckmaier, R.M., Van der Werf, J.T.N., Korte, S.M., Macuhova, J., Korte-Bouws, G., and van Reenen, C.G. (2002) Stress responses during milking; comparing conventional and automatic milking in primiparous dairy cows. *Journal of Dairy Science* 85, 3206–3216.

Leslie, K.E. and Petersson-Wolfe, C.S. (2012) Assessment and management of pain in dairy cows with clinical mastitis. *Veterinary Clinics of North America: Food Animal Practice* 28, 289–305.

Pastell, M., Takko, H., Gröhn, H., Hautala, M., Poikalainen, V., Praks, J., Veermäe, I., Kujala, M. and Ahokas, J. (2006) Assessing cows' welfare: weighing the cow in a milking robot. *Biosystems Engineering* 93, 81–87.

Rousing, T., Bonde, M., Badsberg, J.H. and Sørensen, J.T. (2004) Stepping and kicking behaviour during milking in relation to response in human–animal interaction test and clinical health in loose housed dairy cows. *Livestock Production Science* 88, 1–8.

Rushen, J., de Passillé, A.M. and Munksgaard, L. (1999) Fear of people by cows and effects on milk yield, behaviour and heart rate at milking. *Journal of Dairy Science* 82, 720–727.

Rushen, J., de Passillé, A.M., von Keyserlingk, M.A.G. and Weary, D.M. (2008) *The Welfare of Cattle,* 1st edn. Springer, Dordrecht, The Netherlands.

Rushen, J., Munksgaard, L., Marnet, P.G. and de Passillé, A.M. (2001) Human contact and the effects of acute stress on cows at milking. *Applied Animal Behaviour Science* 73, 1–14.

Siivonen, J., Taponen, S., Hovinen, M., Pastell, M., Lensink, B.J., Pyörälä, S. and Hänninen, L. (2011) Impact of acute clinical mastitis on cow behaviour. *Applied Animal Behaviour Science* 132, 101–106.

CHAPTER 8

Welfare at drying-off and during the dry period

Drying-off is defined as the cessation of milking in lactating dairy cows. The dry period is an important resting period before their next lactation, and the average duration of this period is 40–60 days.

Drying-off in dairy cows implies the gradual or abrupt cessation of milking. Gradual cessation of milking is achieved by reducing the cows' energy intake or frequency of milking before drying-off. Abrupt or sudden drying-off is a common way of stopping milk production at the end of lactation on commercial dairy farms. It involves the cessation of milking without any intended variation in milk production prior to that moment. This means that there is no change in the quantity and quality of feed provided, water availability, or frequency of milking of cows that are still producing significant quantities of milk, perhaps 20–35 kg/day.

The dry period is critically important for the welfare of dairy cows and their production in the following lactation. The main welfare problems

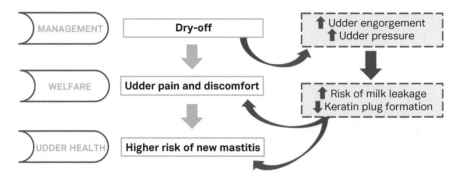

Figure 8.1 Some of the main welfare problems during the dry period in high-producing dairy cows.

during the dry period are pain and discomfort due to udder engorgement, an increased risk of intramammary infections (hereafter called mastitis), restriction of feed and water provision, and aggressive interactions between cows. Figure 8.1 summarizes some of these problems.

> *'Drying-off is a painful and stressful period.'*

Drying-off causes physiological stress. The pain caused by high intramammary pressure after drying-off, particularly if it is abrupt, is accompanied by a stress response. In addition, drying-off is usually associated with several management practices that could act as additional stressors. For example, the cows are usually moved to a different pen and regrouped with other cows, and changed to a low-energy diet. It is worth remembering that stress is additive and that the risk of developing mastitis increases with the stress response.

Physiological changes in the udder at drying-off

At drying-off, the mammary gland continues to produce and secrete milk, resulting in an increased intramammary pressure that may cause pain and stress to the cow. The milk accumulates in the alveoli and ducts of the mammary gland, resulting in udder distension by 16 h after drying-off. Subsequently, there is a degeneration of secretory cells and a disruption of the alveolar and lobular structures of the udder. Around 16–18 h after drying-off, the intramammary pressure rises rapidly, and leakage of milk and a mild inflammatory response occur. Evidence of inflammation includes a transient increase in blood flow in the udder, increased neutrophil counts in milk, and increased permeability of the udder through impairment of tight junctions between the alveolar cells. Intramammary pressure peaks 2 days after drying-off and then decreases, but is present for up to 6 d following abrupt drying-off.

8.1 Pain and discomfort caused by udder engorgement at drying-off

8.1.1 Factors affecting pain and discomfort at drying-off

Drying-off results in the accumulation of a large volume of milk in the udder, leading to udder engorgement, increased pressure, discomfort, and pain. Three main factors affect the pain associated with drying-off.

- **High milk production**. Cows producing higher quantities of milk at drying-off (> 20 kg/day) have larger volumes of mammary secretion during early involution than cows producing less milk (< 15 kg/day). Currently, drying-off on commercial dairy farms involves the cessation of milking in cows that are still producing significant quantities of milk, typically 20–35 kg/day and in some cases as much as 50 kg/day. The risk of discomfort associated with udder engorgement at drying-off is higher in high-producing cows.

- **Abrupt cessation of milking**. Abrupt drying-off with sudden cessation of milking at 40–60 days before the expected calving date is a common management practice. This abrupt form of drying-off causes more pain than a gradual decrease of the milking frequency. In terms of animal welfare, it is preferable to decrease the milking frequency several days before drying-off, to reduce the milk yield. Based on the existing literature, a target milk yield of 15 kg/day or less at drying-off is recommended.
- **Parity**. Primiparous cows can experience more discomfort at drying-off than multiparous cows. Besides their lack of previous experience, primiparous cows have a more persistent milk production curve and a relative immaturity of the mammary gland, which may reduce their tolerance to high intramammary pressure.

8.1.2 Indicators of pain and discomfort at drying-off

There are two main behavioural indicators that can be used to identify cows suffering from udder pain. First, cows reduce their lying time, probably to relieve pressure on the udder. Second, the cows show avoidance behaviour in response to udder palpation.

Reduced lying time

A reduction in lying time can be used as an indicator of discomfort caused by udder distension due to milk accumulation. It has been demonstrated that cows reduce their lying time as a result of udder pain, probably to relieve pressure on the udder. For instance, in one study (O'Driscoll et al., 2011), a reduction in milking frequency from twice to once a day in mid-lactation increased the intramammary pressure and milk leakage, and led to a reduction in the cows' lying behaviour. After milking was omitted, all cows spent more time standing in the resting area instead of lying.

When milking is abruptly stopped in cows with average milk production below 10 kg/day, lying time is not reduced 1 day after drying-off, as their udder firmness increases minimally. However, cows producing on average more than 20 kg/day show a reduction in their lying time, with an increase in the frequency of lying bouts and a decrease in their duration, 1 day after drying-off, which may be indicative of physical discomfort. Given that lying is a high-priority behaviour in dairy cattle (see section 4.1.1), the welfare of cows may be compromised after abrupt milk cessation.

'Reduced lying time at drying-off is indicative of udder pain.'

Behavioural response to udder manipulation

Assessing the reaction of animals to part of their body being manipulated is a commonly used method to assess pain, and is valid and reliable as long as the reaction is scored in a standardized way. Pain sensitivity has been quantified using mechanical (algometers) or thermal (CO_2 laser) stimulation of a hind leg or the udder. These methods measure the nociceptive threshold, defined as the minimum stimulus necessary to elicit a pain response. When a stimulus is applied to a painful site, a cow responds with avoidance behaviours such as kicking, leg lifting, or tail flicking. Lower nociceptive threshold values indicate that there is increased pain. These methods have been used in dairy cows to assess pain associated with lameness or mastitis.

Recently, a score has been described for assessing pain due to udder engorgement in dry cows. Cows are classified into four categories (0 = no udder pain, 1 = light udder pain, 2 = moderate udder pain, and 3 = severe udder pain) depending on their reaction to udder palpation (from no behavioural response to strong avoidance behaviour in response to palpation). Evidence indicates that many cows show signs of pain when their udder is touched shortly after drying off. There is evidence indicating that around 20% of cows suffer pain as a result of udder engorgement in the 2 days following drying-off, and this percentage decreases to 10% on days 3 and 4 after drying-off.

8.1.3 Methods of measuring udder engorgement and udder pressure

Several measures of udder engorgement and/or udder pressure have been suggested as indirect measures of udder pain.

- Udder pressure can be measured using a mechanical stimulus applied to the udder or by palpating the udder.
- The distance between the teats before the last milking, compared with the distance on the following day after drying-off, is useful to assess udder engorgement.
- Leakage of milk from the mammary gland is defined as milk dropping or flowing from any teat, and is a risk factor for mastitis.
- Increased vocalization might be indicative of pain due to udder engorgement, as well as periods of distress or hunger at drying-off.

8.2 Increased risk of mastitis

Several studies have shown that over 60% of new mastitis cases occur during the dry period, and most of them are caused by environmental pathogens. There are two phases within the dry period when susceptibility to a new occurrence of mastitis is particularly high: shortly after drying-off and just before calving.

Several factors increase the risk of new mastitis. Once milking stops, there is neither a flushing of bacteria from the streak canal at each milking nor protection provided by teat dipping. As explained above, udder engorgement due to the abrupt cessation of milking at drying-off may cause milk leakage, and also delays the formation of the keratin plug, and results in the widening and shortening of the streak canal. In addition, milk is a perfect substrate for bacterial growth.

Shortly before calving, susceptibility to infection increases because the keratin plug breaks down, leukocyte function is impaired, and there is leakage of colostrum in some cows. Mastitis is a major welfare problem mainly because it causes pain (see Section 5.3.2).

8.3 Restricted access to feed and water at drying-off

Restriction of feed and water intake is sometimes used as a method to stop milk production. Abrupt restriction of feed and water intake has been associated with stress. Restriction of feed intake represents a metabolic challenge to cattle that results in higher blood concentrations of non-esterified fatty acids, as well as probable hunger and distress, which may be demonstrated by behaviours such as increased vocalization.

8.4 Aggressive interactions and competition between dry cows

As calving approaches, cows are likely to be moved to a new pen and mixed with other cows. Regrouping may occur several times during the last weeks of pregnancy. Regrouping reduces the time cows spend ruminating and increases aggression among them.

Individual cows respond differently to regrouping and this may have important effects on their health status after calving. For example, cows that develop metritis and ketosis after calving have been shown to spend less time feeding during the pre-calving period than cows that remain healthy after calving. Subordinate cows may be particularly at risk, as they are more likely to be driven away from the feed bunk by more dominant cows. Therefore, providing enough feeding space is particularly important to reduce the negative effects of competition between cows.

8.5 Recommendations on husbandry and pain management

Despite the evidence showing that drying-off may have a negative effect on animal welfare, there are very few known practical strategies to reduce welfare problems at drying-off. Because management conditions and facilities vary among farms, farmers and veterinarians should develop individualized protocols for drying-off, always remembering the importance of a clean, dry, comfortable environment for dry cows. Additionally, the following recommendations should be considered.

1. Dry cows are usually allocated to pastures or dry lots to promote exercise during the dry period. It is recommended that these cows have access to a bedded pack and a paved alley, including a resting area equivalent to 10 m²/cow. Bedding material should be removed on a regular basis (preferably daily). In any case, dry cows should be protected from extreme draughts and provided with a dry area to rest for as many hours of the day as they desire.

2. Minimize situations that are likely to cause chronic stress, such as competition for food or water. Ideally, pens should include a feeding trough long enough for all cows to feed at the same time (with a minimum length of 0.76 m of feeder/cow), and each pen should have at least two effective water points.

3. Dry cows should be monitored after drying-off. Identifying milk leakage, palpating the udder, and checking for signs of udder pain can be useful to estimate the incidence of welfare problems related to drying-off.

4. Dry cows should be kept as far as possible from the milking parlour, because the sight, sound, and smell of the parlour will stimulate the milk let-down reflex, resulting in shorter lying periods.

5. A target milk yield of 15 kg/day or less at drying-off is recommended. A 5–7 day period of intermittent milking (e.g. one milking/day)

prior to drying-off, implemented with or without changes in feeding, will lower the milk yield adequately to accelerate involution of the mammary tissue and enhance udder health and cow welfare.

6. In view of the naturally diminishing milk production at weaning when the offspring's need for milk declines, it has recently been proposed to reduce the volume of milk removed at each milking, without altering the frequency of milking, before drying-off of cows with healthy udders. It is expected that increasing the portion of residual milk in the udder in this way will initiate the involution of the mammary tissue. Although applied research on the subject is needed, this gentle preparation for drying-off could contribute to improving the welfare and health of dairy cows.

7. An alternative method to facilitate drying-off is to induce a decrease in milk yield by reducing the level of galactopoietic hormones, such as prolactin, in the blood. For example, cabergoline, a prolactin-release inhibitor that acts at the level of the pituitary gland, reduces blood prolactin concentrations for up to 8 days after administration. However, pharmaceutical products to reduce milk yield at drying-off are generally not available commercially.

Bibliography

Agenäs, S., Dahlborn, K. and Holtenius, K. (2003) Changes in metabolism and milk production during and after feed deprivation in primiparous cows selected for different milk fat content. *Livestock Production Science* 83, 153–164.

Bach, A., De-Prado, A. and Aris, A. (2015) Short communication: The effects of cabergoline administration at dry-off of lactating cows on udder engorgement, milk leakages, and lying behaviour. *Journal of Dairy Science* 98, 7097–7101.

Bachman, K.C. and Schairer, M.L. (2003) Invited review: Bovine studies on optimal lengths of dry periods. *Journal of Dairy Science* 86, 3027–3037.

Bertulat, S., Fischer-Tenhagen, C., Suthar, V., Möstl, E., Isaka, N. and Heuwieser, W. (2013) Measurement of fecal glucocorticoid metabolites and evaluation of udder characteristics to estimate stress after sudden dry-off in dairy cows with different milk yields. *Journal of Dairy Science* 96, 3774–3787.

Boutinaud, M., Isaka, N., Lollivier, V., Dessauge, F., Gandemer, E., Lamberton, P., De Prado Taranilla, A.I., Deflandre, A. and Sordillo, L.M. (2016) Cabergoline inhibits prolactin secretion and accelerates involution in dairy cows after dry-off. *Journal of Dairy Science* 99, 5707–5718.

Chapinal, N., Zobel, G., Painter, K. and Leslie, K.E. (2014) Changes in lying behaviour after abrupt cessation of milking and regrouping at dry-off in freestall-housed cows: A case study. *Journal of Veterinary Behavior* 9, 364–369.

Davis, S.R., Farr, V.C. and Stelwagen, K. (1999) Regulation of yield loss and milk composition during once-daily milking: a review. *Livestock Production Science* 59, 77–94.

Dingwell, R.T., Leslie, K.E., Schukken, Y.H., Sargeant, J.M., Timms, L.L., Duffield, T.F., Keefe, G.P., Kelton, D.F., Lissemore, K.D. and Conklin, J. (2004) Association of cow and quarter-level factors at drying-off with new intramammary infections during the dry period. *Preventive Veterinary Medicine* 63, 75–89.

Ledgerwood, D.N., Winckler, C. and Tucker, C.B. (2010) Evaluation of data loggers, sampling intervals, and editing techniques for measuring the lying behavior of dairy cattle. *Journal of Dairy Science* 93, 5129–5139.

Martin, L.M., Sauerwein, H., Büscher, W. and Müller, U. (2020) Automated gradual reduction of milk yield before dry-off: effects on udder health, involution and inner teat morphology. *Livestock Science* 233, 103942.

Metz, J.H.M. (1985) The reaction of cows to a short-term deprivation of lying. *Applied Animal Behaviour Science* 13, 301–307.

Odensten, M.O., Berglund, B., Waller, J.P. and Holtenius, K. (2007) Metabolism and udder health at dry-off in cows of different breeds and production levels. *Journal of Dairy Science* 90, 1417–1428.

O'Driscoll, K., Gleeson, D., O'Brien, B. and Boyle, L. (2011) Does omission of a regular milking event affect cow comfort? *Livestock Science* 138, 132–143.

Österman, S. and Redbo, I. (2001) Effects of milking frequency on lying down and getting up behavior in dairy cows. *Applied Animal Behaviour Science* 70, 167–176.

Steeneveld, W., de Prado-Taranilla, A., Krogh, K. and Hogeveen, H. (2018) The economic impact of drying off cows with a dry-off facilitator (cabergoline) compared with 2 methods of gradual cessation of lactation for European dairy farms. *Journal of Dairy Science* 102, 7483–7493.

Tucker, C.B., Lacy-Hulbert, S.J. and Webster, J.R. (2009) Effect of milking frequency and feeding level before and after dry off on dairy cattle behavior and udder characteristics. *Journal of Dairy Science* 92, 3194–3203.

Vilar, M.J. and Rajala-Schultz, P.J. (2020) Dry-off and dairy cow udder health and welfare: Effects of different milk cessation methods. *The Veterinary Journal* 262, 105503.

Zobel, G., Weary, D.M., Leslie, K.E. and von Keyserlingk, M.A.G. (2015) Invited review: Cessation of lactaion: effects on animal welfare. *Journal of Dairy Science* 98, 8263–8277.

CHAPTER 9

Welfare during the peripartum period

A normal calving (eutocia) poses a risk for both the mother and the newborn calf. In the case of a difficult calving (dystocia), this risk is greater. Management during the peripartum period can be critical to the mother's health, and the effects of good management can last into the next lactation period. Perinatal mortality accounts for half of all deaths of calves before weaning. Thus, the peripartum period involves both welfare issues and potential economic loss, both of which can be mitigated by improving the management of animals during this period.

9.1 Calving is a painful and stressful process

It is generally accepted that giving birth causes acute pain in all species, including cattle. Around the time of birth, the levels of acute phase proteins such as haptoglobin and serum amyloid protein increase considerably in response to inflammation and tissue damage, and, thus, pain. Dystocia can cause intense pain not only in the mother, but also in the calf.

Any calving also causes physiological stress. Calving is associated with increased plasma cortisol concentrations irrespective of the parturition environment. The reasons for this are twofold: first, pain is always accompanied by a stress response and, second, any new or uncommon situation can trigger stress.

The pain and stress caused by calving are important not only because of their negative impact on animal welfare, but also because they can have significant consequences for the entire birth process, as they inhibit the release of oxytocin, and can therefore decrease myometrial contractions and delay the secretion of colostrum.

9.2 Behavioural changes during normal calving

The process of calving has been divided into three stages:

- **stage I** – from dilation of the cervix to the expulsion of amniotic fluid
- **stage II** – from the expulsion of amniotic fluid to the expulsion of the calf
- **stage III** – from the expulsion of the calf to the expulsion of the placenta.

It is important to be familiar with the normal behavioural changes during calving in order to recognize problematic births. The characteristics of stages I and II of a normal calving are summarized in Table 9.1.

In stage III (from the expulsion of the calf until the expulsion of the placenta), uterine contractions persist, decreasing in amplitude but becoming more frequent and less regular. Normal expulsion of the placenta occurs within 8 h after delivery of the calf. Retained placenta is defined as the failure to void fetal membranes within 24 h. During this stage, the dam begins to lick the calf.

Parturition begins gradually, which often makes it difficult to tell exactly when it has begun. In practice, raising and arching the tail is one of the

Table 9.1 Characteristics of normal calving: stages I and II.

	Stage I	Stage II
Description	From dilation of the cervix to expulsion of amniotic fluid	From expulsion of amniotic fluid to expulsion of the calf
Approximate duration	4 h	60–100 min
Normal behaviours	Decreased food intake and rumination Restlessness Increased exploratory behaviour Frequent changes in posture Looking at own flanks, kicking, scraping the ground, raising and arching the tail	Lying on side or remaining in a resting position
Contractions	Uterine Abdominal (initially irregular; by the end, coming at 15 min intervals and lasting 20 s)	Abdominal (regular, coming every 3 min and lasting 30 s)

most valuable indicators of imminent calving (Figure 9.1). The highest frequencies of tail-up behaviour are observed before calving, and this behaviour is seen earlier in heifers, from 4 h before calving, compared with 2 h before calving in cows. Currently, different types of devices for calving detection are on the market, which could predict the onset of calving several hours in advance. These include, for instance, inclinometers that detect tail raising, accelerometers that detect restlessness, abdominal belts that monitor uterine contractions, vaginal probes that detect a decrease in vaginal temperature, and collars that can detect a combination of increases in bouts of lying and decreases in rumination chews.

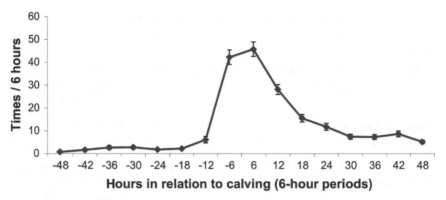

Figure 9.1 Frequency of tail-up behaviour (means +/- standard error) in relation to time around calving (reprinted from *Journal of Veterinary Behavior*, 9(6), Eva Mainau, Anna Cuevas, José LuisRuiz-de-la-Torre, Elke Abbeloos, Xavier Manteca, Effect of meloxicam administration after calving on milk production, acute phase proteins, and behavior in dairy cows, 357–363, Copyright (2014), with permission from Elsevier).

9.3 Difficult calving

In cows, calving usually lasts between 30 min and 4 h from the time the amnion begins to protrude through the vulva to the expulsion of the calf. Dystocia refers to difficult birth due to either a prolonged spontaneous parturition or a severe (requiring the application of force by ropes or a mechanical device to pull the calf) or prolonged assisted extraction. It is associated with unacceptably high levels of pain.

Many studies have shown that calving difficulties occur at a low incidence (from 2% to 5%). However, it has also been reported that as many as 50% of calvings are assisted on some Swiss dairy farms, and that 24% of calvings in the USA involved dystocia. In the UK, it is reported that 8.7% of calvings are assisted, although this proportion varied from 0% to 57% across farms. This huge variability among countries and farms is probably due to the variation in identifying calvings that need assistance. In fact, this is not an easy task, as there is no standardized scale for measuring calving difficulty; additionally, more objective measures are needed to help determine when assistance is truly beneficial.

Different scales have been developed to score the degree of calving difficulty. The force required to deliver the calf is one proposed way for use in the field (Table 9.2 and Figure 9.2).

Table 9.2 Example of a calving difficulty scale.

Score	Definition
1	No assistance
2	Easy pull by hand
3	Hard pull by ropes
4	Hard pull by mechanical calf puller
5	Caesarean section

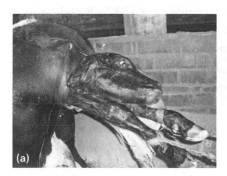 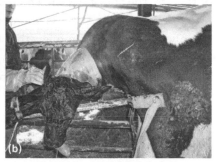

Figure 9.2 Difficult extraction (a) by ropes and (b) by a mechanical calf puller due to disproportion between the size of the fetus and the diameter of the dam's pelvis.

'Dystocia refers to a difficult birth due to either a prolonged spontaneous parturition or a severe or prolonged assisted extraction. It is associated with unacceptably high levels of pain.'

The two main causes of dystocia in cows are disproportion between the size of the calf and the diameter of the pelvis (more common in heifers) and malpresentation of the calf (more common in multiparous cows).

In general, dystocia is more frequent in heifers than in multiparous cows, and delivery for a heifer is believed to be more painful and stressful. This is due not only to the heifer's lack of experience, but also to the fact that calving tends to take longer in heifers than in multiparous cows. The degree of effort associated with calving is usually greater in heifers than in multiparous cows, especially during the early processes of calving (stage I). Calving in heifers is also accompanied by a more pronounced inflammatory response and a slower postpartum recovery compared with that of multiparous cows.

A Caesarean section (CS) is potentially indicated in cases of dystocia in order to reduce the probability of death of the cow and/or calf. Calf malpresentation is the main reason for veterinarians to perform a CS. Calf malpresentation is influenced by the presence of twins, the breed of the sire, the sex of the calf (males have twice the risk as females), and fetal mortality. The success rate of CS and its impact on animal welfare mainly depends on the operative technique. In a CS, the use of local anaesthesia (procaine or lidocaine), alpha-2-agonists (such as xylazine), and a non-steroidal anti-inflammatory drug (NSAID) is needed to control pain.

9.3.1 Behavioural changes during difficult calving

Recent studies suggest that some behavioural traits could be used as predictors of difficult calving or, at least, calving requiring human assistance. The possibility of dystocia should be considered if any stage of the calving is excessively prolonged, if atypical behaviour is observed at a given stage, or if changes are observed in the frequency of otherwise normal behaviours.

Stage I (from dilation of the cervix to expulsion of amniotic fluid)

A drastic reduction in food intake is one indicator of dystocia. The activity of cows increases quite dramatically prior to parturition. It has been suggested that this increased restlessness may be due to discomfort, but this behaviour might also be a part of the normal calving situation. An increased frequency of certain behaviours, such as changes in posture, kicking, scraping the ground, rubbing against the wall, or raising the tail for longer before calving, is likewise an indicator of dystocia.

Stage II (from expulsion of amniotic fluid to expulsion of the calf)

In normal calvings, the abdominal contractions are often interrupted, providing some rest. Longer abdominal contractions and higher frequency of contractions are associated with dystocia. In dystocic calvings, a high percentage of cows will stand before this stage is completed.

Stage III (from expulsion of the calf to expulsion of the placenta)

An association between difficult parturition and delayed standing of the dam after parturition has been reported in cows. Nevertheless, more research is needed in this area, because the management practice of placing the newborn calf in front of the dam following an assisted delivery may contribute to longer periods of recumbency. The degree of difficulty of the calving is reflected in the newborn's behaviour, as calves will take longer to stand up and to begin nursing after a difficult birth.

Vocalizations can be useful welfare indicators in conditions involving pain. However, vocalizations during parturition are not always present, perhaps as an adaptation to avoid attracting predators. Moreover, it must be taken into account that vocal responses show great individual variability and can indicate states other than pain, such as hunger, isolation, separation, or fear.

9.4 Health and productive consequences of calving

Parturition is an intrinsically risky process for both the mother and the offspring. The injury, trauma, and inflammation associated with parturition (particularly in dystocia) can have important negative effects on the health and productivity of dairy cows, and their effects can extend into the following lactation.

9.4.1 Consequences for the cow

A reduction in food and water intake and consequent weight loss are commonly seen in cows after calving, especially in heifers. Cows that experience partum and postpartum disorders (e.g. dystocia, retained placenta, or parturient paresis) have been found to reduce their dry matter intake by 20% after calving. Increasing cows' food intake after parturition can minimize metabolic disorders and weight loss, and improve their reproductive performance.

Feed intake and milk production are closely related. Cows with a higher body condition score at calving produced more milk, containing higher levels of fat and protein, in the first 90 days of lactation. Dystocic calving significantly reduced milk production and milk fat and protein content. In addition, milk production was reduced by an estimated 12% of the potential yield in cows that needed a CS at parturition.

Health problems peak around parturition in cows. Around 10% of cows have recto-vaginal injuries after calving. The risk factors for such injuries are parity (heifers have a higher risk than multiparous cows), male calves, and dystocic calvings. In some cases, recto-vaginal injuries lead to faecal contamination, which may result in endometritis, which in turn can lead to lower fertility. Other possible consequences of calving, especially dystocic calvings, are vulval discharges, metritis, and retained placenta. Maternal mortality also peaks around parturition in cows. Cow deaths increase by about 4% for all parity groups in cows with very difficult calvings, compared with cows needing no assistance at calving.

9.4.2 Consequences for the calf

Prolonged or difficult deliveries (without a CS) are associated with increased calf mortality. For instance, malpresented calves are five times as likely as normally presented calves to be stillborn. Perinatal mortality in calves ranges from 4% to 13%, and half of all pre-weaning deaths occur within the first day of life. Newborns requiring assistance at parturition might develop a severe acidosis because of oxygen deprivation, with subsequent effects on the function of vital organs and overall vitality. Reduced vigour, poor thermoregulation, failure of passive transfer of maternal immunity via colostrum intake, poor performance, and greater susceptibility to infections are also important secondary problems associated with neonatal asphyxia and acidosis.

9.5 Prevention and management recommendations

Controllable factors such as the breed or strain of the sire and dam, maternal feeding, and maternal body condition score at calving are important aspects to consider in order to reduce the risk of dystocia due to a disproportion between the size of the calf and the diameter of the dam's pelvis. For instance, different strategies for maternal feeding can avoid the adverse effect of under- or over-feeding during the last trimester of pregnancy, which can affect birth weight and the deposition of adipose tissue in the birth canal, with consequent increased risk of dystocia and stillbirth.

It is important to minimize situations liable to cause chronic stress, such as competition for food, water, or a place to lie down. Ideally, prepartum pens should include a resting area equivalent to 11 m²/cow and a feeding area big enough for all cows to feed at the same time (minimum of 0.76 m length of feeder/cow). Additionally, each pen should have at least two water points.

The cow should be monitored once an hour from the onset of stage I of calving without disturbing her. Intervention is necessary only if any stage of the calving process is excessively protracted and/or if atypical behaviour, or normal behaviour with an abnormal frequency, is observed.

Individual calving stalls should be arranged so that the cows within can make eye contact with other cows. This arrangement enables efficient monitoring of calving by the stockperson, as well as proper expression of maternal behaviours in postparturient dams. Individual stalls should have a surface area of at least 12 m², be provided with straw bedding, and be hygienic.

Group calving pens should never hold more than 25 cows each and should be designed to allow cows in labour to be separated without having to be removed from the pen. To facilitate this, a mobile barrier inside the group calving pen is recommended. Be aware that separated areas inside the group calving pen should be clean (Figure 9.3) and should have water available.

Moving cows too early to an individual calving stall (or to a separated area inside the calving pen) will affect the cleanliness of the calving environment. If cows spend 3 or more days in the maternity unit, they are at greater risk for elevated blood concentrations of non-esterified fatty acids, ketosis, and displaced abomasum. It is recommended to move cows to the maternity unit within 1 or 2 days prior to their expected date of calving in order to provide an adequate environment for calving and to detect abnormal calving early. However, as it can be difficult to predict this pre-calving time accurately, it may be preferable to move

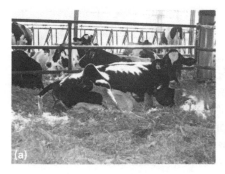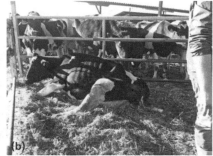

Figure 9.3 Examples of a separated area inside a group calving pen: (a) clean; (b) dirty.

cows that have already initiated calving (stage II) than to move cows that are about to start calving (stage I). It is likely that any environmental disturbance that occurs when the cow is moved may reduce or inhibit uterine contractions if initiated in stage I of calving, but will cause only a temporary decrease in uterine motility if initiated in stage II of calving.

Dams should be allowed to lick and ingest the amniotic fluid on the calf. Not only does this behaviour increase the calf's vigour, it also helps to reduce the pain caused by the calving in the dam because the amniotic fluid contains certain compounds that enhance the analgesic action of endogenous opioids.

In the peripartum period, the use of palliative pain treatments should be considered. The administration of an NSAID following calving can reduce pain and inflammation, improve the cow's health and welfare, and help to maintain or increase fertility and milk yield. Scientific data on the impact of analgesics following calving are, however, limited and often contradictory.

Cow–calf separation after calving

Concern from the public is growing regarding early cow–calf separation after calving. The effects of early separation versus extended cow–calf contact on the behaviour of cows and calves are mixed, and the variables measured to date make it difficult to draw strong conclusions about overall welfare. Early separation (within 24 h postpartum) reduces the acute distress responses of cows and calves. Nevertheless, longer cow–calf contact typically has positive longer-term effects on calves, promoting more normal social behaviour, reducing abnormal behaviour, and sometimes reducing responses to stressors. In terms of productivity, allowing cows to nurse calves decreased the volume of milk available for sale during the nursing period, but there is no consistent evidence of reduced milk production over a longer period. Allowing a prolonged period of nursing increased calf weight gain during the milk-feeding period. In addition, prolonged cow–calf contact has documented health benefits for calves, namely, increased immunoglobulin absorption from colostrum, and decreased mortality rates. Still, studies on the long-term effects of dam rearing on behaviour, udder health, and farm economics are few.

In practice, the following free-contact cow–calf systems may be a viable option for some producers, even in modern dairy systems.

- Free-contact systems where the cow and calf have unrestricted access to each other.
- Restricted sucking systems allowing a short period of contact daily only to nurse.
- Half-day contact where the cow and calf are housed together during the day or night.
- Foster cow systems where one cow nurses two to four calves, usually without also being milked.

These free-contact cow–calf systems originate, to a large extent, from practical developments and the experience of farmers who keep cows and calves together (e.g. organic dairy farmers in Norway and Sweden).

Additional research is needed to determine whether these systems are practical options in modern dairy systems. There are several drawbacks that need to be addressed: for example, management practices for welfare-friendly weaning, how to establish a good human–calf relationship with calves that are nursed, how to improve the milking procedure for nursing cows, and how to control potential transmissible or contagious diseases in cattle kept in mixed age groups.

Bibliography

Barrier, A.C., Haskell, M.J., Macrae, A.I. and Dwyer, C.M. (2012) Parturition progress and behaviours in dairy cows with calving difficulty. *Applied Animal Behaviour Science* 139, 209–217.

Beaver, A., Meagher, R.K., von Keyserlingk, M.A.G. and Weary, D.M. (2019) Invited review: A systematic review of the effects of early separation on dairy cow and calf health. *Journal of Dairy Science* 102, 5784–5810.

Cook, N.B. and Nordlund, K.V. (2004) Behavioral needs of the transition cow and considerations for special needs facility design. *Veterinary Clinics of North America: Food Animal Practice* 20, 495–520.

Johnsen, J.F., Zipp, K.A., Kälber, T., de Passillé, A.M., Knicrim, U., Barth, K. and Mejdell, C.M. (2016) Is rearing calves with the dam a feasible option for dairy farms?—Current and future research. *Applied Animal Behaviour Science* 181, 1-11.

Kolkman, I., Aerts, S., Vervaecke, H., Vicca, J., Vandelook, J., de Kruif, A., Opsomer, G. and Lips, D. (2008) Assessment of differences in some indicators of pain in double muscled Belgian Blue cows following naturally calving vs. Caesarean section. *Reproduction in Domestic Animals* 45, 160–167.

Laven, R., Chambers, P. and Stafford, K. (2012) Using non-steroidal anti-inflammatory drugs around calving: maximizing comfort, productivity and fertility. *The Veterinary Journal* 192, 8–12.

Mahmoud, F., Christopher, B., Maher, A., Jürg, H., Alexander, S., Adrian, S. and Gaby, H. (2017) Prediction of calving time in dairy cattle. *Animal Reproduction Science* 187, 37–46.

Mainau, E., Cuevas, A., Ruiz-de-la-Torre, J.L., Abbeloos, E. and Manteca, X. (2014) Effect of meloxicam administration after calving on milk production, acute phase proteins, and behaviour in dairy cows. *Journal of Veterinary Behavior* 9, 357–363.

Mainau, E. and Manteca, X. (2011) Pain and discomfort caused by parturition in cows and sows. *Applied Animal Behaviour Science* 135, 241–251.

Meagher, R.K., Beaver, A., Weary, D.M. and von Keyserlingk, M.A.G. (2019) Invited review: A systematic review of the effects of prolonged cow–calf contact on behaviour, welfare and productivity. *Journal of Dairy Science* 102, 5765-5783.

Mee, J.F. (2008) Prevalence and risk factors for dystocia in dairy cattle: a review. *The Veterinary Journal* 176, 93–101.

Qu, Y., Fadden, A.N., Traber, M.G. and Bobe, G. (2014) Potential risk indicators of retained placenta and other diseases in multiparous cows. *Journal of Dairy Science* 97, 4151–4165.

Saint-Dizier, M. and Chastant-Maillard, S. (2018) Methods and on-farm devices to predict calving time in cattle. *The Veterinary Journal* 205, 349–356.

CHAPTER 10

Welfare of calves until weaning

Dairy calves are exposed to a series of challenges straight after their birth. They are separated from their mothers and usually kept individually in hutches until they are weaned and transferred to large groups. During this period, many factors will challenge calves in many areas that have an impact on their welfare, including nutrition, comfort, health, and their emotional state.

10.1 Importance of sucking behaviour

Sucking is a **natural behaviour** that calves are highly motivated to perform. If a natural behaviour such as sucking cannot be performed, calves show a stress response, which can be identified by the expression of abnormal behaviours.

In natural conditions, calves suck in several episodes of approximately 6–12 min, distributed throughout the day. Sucking increases the release of enzymes (e.g. renin and pepsin) and hormones (e.g. insulin and cholecystokinin) that are important for digestion. In addition, sucking stimulates the closure of the oesophageal groove, which ensures milk goes directly to the abomasum; this prevents the milk from reaching the rumen and causing abnormal fermentation that increases the risk of diarrhoea. By contrast, if milk is provided from a bucket, calves spend no more than approximately 1 min to drink the milk. For this reason, straight after taking milk from a bucket, some calves show a redirected sucking behaviour: they suck parts of the body of other calves or the pen facilities, reproducing the same movements as in sucking. These behaviours are indicative of a welfare deficiency that may be associated with either the impossibility to suck or the provision of small quantities of milk, or both. Feeding calves via an artificial nipple or teat rather than a bucket or providing them with a non-nutritive artificial teat following a milk meal may prevent these cross-sucking behaviours.

10.2 Problems related to housing

Calves are usually separated from their mothers early on after calving and kept individually in small hutches that prevent contact with other calves. The reason for this isolation is that calves kept in groups or with close contact to other calves may develop cross-sucking behaviours that are considered problematic or can injuriously affect their herd-mates, such as navel or teat sucking or urine drinking. In addition, it is thought that group housing may facilitate the transmission of disease from sick calves. Nevertheless, rearing calves individually interrupts the development of social behaviour and reduces the expression of other behaviours, such as playing, which is considered an important behaviour for calves.

'Housing calves in small groups of two to four animals shows good benefits in terms of welfare and growth.'

Group housing of calves is based on the principle that dairy cattle are herd animals, and housing calves in groups allows the development of social herd behaviour and interactions. Group housing also provides the opportunity for calves to exercise and play within the group and provides more calf-to-calf contact and enrichment stimulus, compared with individual housing (Figure 10.1). Small groups of calves can be managed successfully, but it is difficult to manage nutrition and control disease in large groups. Large groups of calves (eight to ten animals per group) show a higher incidence of enteric and/or respiratory diseases and higher mortality rates than those housed in smaller groups before

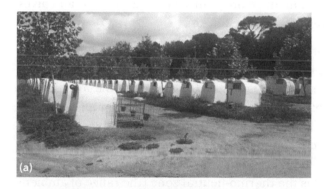

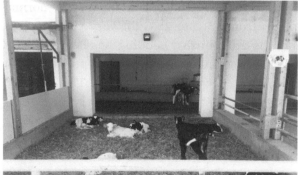

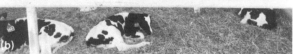

Figure 10.1 Different kinds of calf housing: (a) individual hutches and (b) as a large group with automatic feeding.

weaning. However, calves housed in small groups of two to four animals show improvements in terms of growth and health compared with calves housed either in large groups or individually.

Because calves spend most of their time lying down, the conditions of the resting area are important for the calves' welfare. Spaces for calves must be constructed such that each calf can lie down and stand up, rest, and self-groom without difficulty. Typically, the size of individual hutches for calves until 8 weeks of age varies from 1.2 to 1.5 m width and 2.0 to 2.4 m length. It is recommended that hutches have an outdoor run, preferably of more than 2 m², enabling some contact with other calves. The space required for calves in group pens varies according to their weight. The recommended area ranges from 2 m²/calf (for calves of 45 kg) to 5 m²/calf (for calves of 150 kg).

Bedding is usually provided within the pen to help with moisture control and to aid in maintaining the calves' body temperature in colder environments. Dryness and cleanliness (hygiene) are the most important characteristics of the resting area, and pens for young calves are usually fully bedded. Bedding is important to prevent calves experiencing cold, as cold affects younger, sick, or injured animals much more severely than it does to mature, healthy animals. Thermal comfort for animals is quantified as the thermo-neutral zone (the range of ambient temperatures at which the body temperature is maintained by normal metabolism), which ranges from 15°C to 25°C for very young calves (those in the first 2 months after birth). Bedding has been directly related to the risk of developing pneumonia, and calves provided with an abundant bed of straw show a lower risk of sickness. This could be due to a lower maintenance energy requirement and a better performance of the immune system. Straw and bark chips make good bedding materials for calves, as they are absorbent materials with good insulating properties (Figure 10.2). Fine particles of sawdust and sand are not recommended at all. Sand does not provide any insulating properties and has poor absorbing ability.

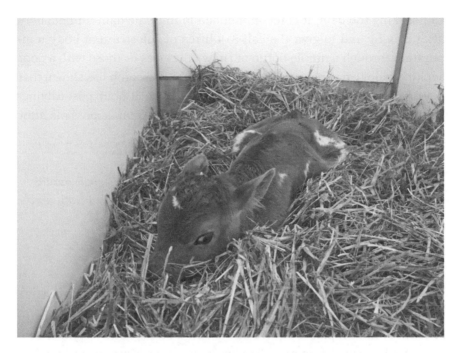

Figure 10.2 Calf bedded in dry straw in order to avoid heat loss.

10.3 Problems related to feeding

10.3.1 Colostrum

Calves require colostrum for disease prevention and nutrition. Colostrum provides a highly digestible source of energy, protein, and antibodies. The ingestion of a sufficient quantity of good-quality colostrum immediately after birth is the most important factor that determines the survival and health of calves. The three key factors for the optimal transfer of maternal immunity via colostrum are the **quality** of the colostrum (in terms of the immunoglobulin G (IgG) concentration), the **amount** ingested, and the efficiency of **absorption** of the IgG within the colostrum by the small intestine. If colostrum is not obtained by the calf sucking the dam, it is recommended to milk the dam immediately after calving and to give the calf 3–4 litres of colostrum at body temperature through a nipple bottle or (in weak calves or those with a poor sucking reflex) via an oesophageal feeder tube. Research has shown that colostral IgG concentration decreases by 3.7% each hour post-calving. For this reason, colostrum should be obtained as soon as possible after calving and never after 6 h post-calving.

> 'The ingestion of a sufficient quantity of colostrum of good quality after birth is the most important factor that determines the health and survival of calves.'

10.3.2 Milk

Traditionally, it has been advised that sucking calves be fed a daily amount of milk replacer equivalent to 10% of their body weight to promote feed consumption and allow early weaning. More recently, it has been recommended to increase the intake of milk replacer to an amount equivalent to 20% of body weight in order to avoid chronic hunger. Feed restriction can have long-lasting consequences for calves. Recent studies suggest that calves that receive a greater amount of milk have a lower incidence of pathologies and produce more milk in their first lactation.

10.3.3 Water

From 2–3 days of age, fresh water should be offered to all calves. Water availability is important in terms of animal welfare to satisfy thirst, and water intake is clearly related to feed consumption and rumen development. Water goes directly into the rumen and creates the ideal environment for fermentation by rumen bacteria. By contrast, milk or milk replacer goes directly into the abomasum and does not contribute to the development of the rumen. In young calves, water consumption has been reported to vary from 0.17 l/day to 1.1 l/day during the first 3 weeks of life, and can be even higher depending on the climate and the calves' health status. For instance, during heat stress or in animals with diarrhoea, water intake can increase by between 25% and 50%. Access to water also reduces cross-sucking behaviours, as water serves as a form of environmental enrichment.

10.3.4 Starter concentrate and fibre

Calves should have access to clean and palatable starter concentrate from 3 days of age onwards. Concentrates should be introduced by placing a small amount in a shallow bucket with the aim of encouraging consumption.

Similarly, fibre may be introduced by day 3 of life, and should be available to all calves by 2 weeks of age. Fibre promotes the growth of the muscular layer of the rumen and helps maintain the health of the rumen lining through its abrasive effect, which prevents papillae clumping together.

Fibre quality is very important for calf performance. Studies have shown that providing pre-weaning calves with chopped forage such as oat or ryegrass hay, triticale silage, and barley straw, separately from the starter concentrate, improves their growth at weaning and is associated with a greater intake of concentrate compared with calves that are not provided with forage and those receiving alfalfa hay. The source of fibre that is fed should, if possible, be different from the bedding, to reduce the likelihood of calves eating contaminated bedding and consuming pathogenic organisms at the same time.

10.4 Problems related to health

The main diseases affecting calves are diarrhoea and pneumonia. Diarrhoea is the main cause of illness during lactation, followed by pneumonia, which becomes the main cause after weaning. Both diseases significantly affect the welfare of calves and can have long-lasting effects, not only on the growth of calves, but also on their future productivity in adulthood. Both diseases are multifactorial; this means that the disease is the result of a combination of numerous factors, in which proper handling and the provision of colostrum play a fundamental role.

Causes of diarrhoea and respiratory disease

The cause of diarrhoea can be infectious or nutritional. Infectious diarrhoea is caused by viruses (rotavirus, coronavirus), bacteria (*Escherichia coli*, *Salmonella* spp.), and parasites (coccidia, *Cryptosporidium parvum*), all of which can act independently or in concert. Nutritional diarrhoea is usually caused by stress due to a breakdown in the management routine related to the administration of milk.

The infectious agents involved in respiratory problems include viruses (respiratory syncytial virus, bovine herpesvirus (the agent of infectious bovine rhinotracheitis)) and bacteria (*Mannheimia haemolytica*, *Pasteurella multocida*, *Mycoplasma bovis*), among others.

10.4.1 Diarrhoea

Neonatal diarrhoea (scour) in calves is characterized by the acute appearance of loose or watery faeces. It affects between 10% and 35% of sucking calves and is responsible for more than 50% of pre-weaning deaths. Diarrhoea causes lethargy and a gradual loss of appetite and growth.

After 1 or 2 days with diarrhoea, calves can become dehydrated and lose between 5% and 12% of their body weight. As the calves become dehydrated, their clinical signs (sunken eyes, low skin elasticity, dry mouth and nose, cold limbs and ears) are more pronounced, and dehydration can cause death.

In calves with diarrhoea, food malabsorption increases the low comfort temperature, meaning that they are more susceptible to cold temperatures. A change in resting behaviour has also been described, at least in small calves, and calves with diarrhoea can be seen more frequently with their limbs under their body and their head resting to one side. Diarrhoea can be accompanied by pain, and calves with diarrhoea often adopt a pain-relieving posture, with a tucked-up abdomen and the tail between the hind legs while they are standing. In addition to these acute changes, several long-term consequences of diarrhoea have been described in replacement heifers, including an increase in the age at first calving and a lower milk production during the first lactation.

Although specific treatments are available for scour, depending on the causal pathogen, in all cases it is important to ensure that calves receive:

- enough liquid and electrolytes to replace those lost in the faeces
- normal amounts of milk or milk replacer for as long as they want to drink it.

10.4.2 Pneumonia

Pneumonia (inflammation of the lungs) is the second most common health problem affecting young calves. Approximately 3% of live-born calves die from pneumonia in the first 3 months of life. Pneumonia is highly infectious, often affecting more than 50% of young calves in a group. Pneumonia is a multifactorial disease, and the main factors involved are presented in Figure 10.3.

Early symptoms of pneumonia are a reduced feed intake or appetite, dullness, fever, and cough. Other later signs may include an increased respiratory rate and nasal or ocular discharge.

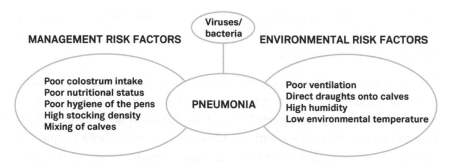

Figure 10.3 Main risk factors for pneumonia in calves.

10.4.3 Prevention and treatment

A number of steps can be taken to help prevent diseases in calves, including diarrhoea and pneumonia.

- Ensure adequate colostrum intake.
- Avoid chronic hunger by offering milk or milk replacement in an amount equivalent to 15–20% of the calves' body weight.
- Allow calves to perform their natural sucking behaviour by using nipples instead of buckets for feeding.
- Calves must have permanent access to clean, fresh water.
- Offer optimal hygienic conditions and well-ventilated housing.
- Minimize stressful conditions such as rough handling, transport, or mixing, as stress may increase the susceptibility of animals to infectious agents.
- Sick animals must be separated from the rest of the group and moved to hospital pens to be treated properly.
- Antibiotics do not work against parasites and viruses. However, where bacterial involvement is suspected, antibiotic treatment is required.
- Vaccination should be considered. If the dams are vaccinated, they will transfer maternal immunity through colostrum (as in the case

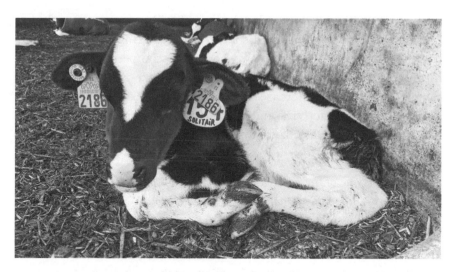

Figure 10.4 Calf with diarrhoea showing sickness behaviour, which includes lethargy, somnolence, decreased activity, and loss of appetite and thirst. The calf's ears are lowered, a sign of pain.

of diarrhoea), or calves themselves can be vaccinated before the period of greatest risk (as in the case of pneumonia at weaning).

- The administration of a non-steroidal anti-inflammatory drug (NSAID) as an effective supportive therapy to reduce discomfort and sickness behaviour is now increasingly being included as part of the treatment of diarrhoea and pneumonia in calves (Figure 10.4).

10.5 Stress at weaning

Weaning is one of the most stressful periods for a calf. Under natural conditions, weaning occurs gradually between 7 and 14 months of age, with the calf progressively increasing the time spent away from the mother and replacing milk with solid feed (forage). By contrast, in intensive conditions, calves are first separated from the mother the first day and then weaned abruptly, usually at between 8 and 12 weeks of age. Stress at the time of weaning is due to the combination of various stressors: nutritional (due to the absence of milk), environmental (due to the change of housing) and social (due to mixing with unfamiliar calves). As a result of the stress response, the competence of the calf's immune system is compromised, and feed intake is decreased; combined, these changes increase the risk of illness. Behavioural changes such as increased activity and vocalizations, and redirected sucking behaviours, are indicators of stress at weaning.

> *'Weaning is one of the most stressful periods for calves, as they have to face nutritional, environmental, and social changes.'*

Stress has an additive effect, so it is recommended to reduce the number of sources of stress in critical periods such as weaning. A practical strategy to decrease the stress response is to perform weaning in two separate phases, progressively removing the milk first and changing the housing pen thereafter. This practice improves the calves' growth and reduces the incidence of respiratory problems. Ideally, calves should be placed in small groups that remain stable from birth onwards.

Gradual weaning may also improve the welfare of calves by allowing them to progressively habituate, over 10–14 days, to the new feed. With this strategy, calves progressively increase their ingestion of solid feed, reducing frustration due to hunger and ultimately decreasing cross-sucking behaviours.

Bibliography

Bach, A., Ahedo, J. and Ferrer, A. (2010) Optimizing weaning strategies of dairy replacement calves. *Journal of Dairy Science* 93, 413–419.

Bernal-Rigoli, J.C., Allen, J.D., Marchello, J.A., Cuneo, S.P., Garcia, S.R., Xie, G., Hall, L.W., Burrows, C.D. and Duff, G.C. (2012) Effects of housing and feeding systems on performance of neonatal Holstein bull calves. *Journal of Animal Science* 90, 2818–2825.

Borderas, T.F., de Passillé, A.M. and Rushen, J. (2009) Feeding behavior of calves fed small or large amounts of milk. *Journal of Dairy Science* 92, 2843–2852.

Bøe, K.E. and Færevik, G. (2003) Grouping and social preferences in calves, heifers and cows. *Applied Animal Behaviour Science* 80, 175–190.

Castells, L., Bach, A., Aris, A. and Terré, M. (2013) Effects of forage provision to young calves on rumen fermentation and development of the gastrointestinal tract. *Journal of Dairy Science* 96, 5226–5236.

Castells, L., Bach, A. and Terré, M. (2015) Short- and long-term effects of forage supplementation of calves during the preweaning period on performance, reproduction, and milk yield at first lactation. *Journal of Dairy Science* 98, 4748–4753.

Costa, J.H.C., von Keyserlingk, M.A.G. and Weary, D.M. (2016) Invited review: Effects of group housing of dairy calves on behavior, cognition, performance, and health. *Journal of Dairy Science* 99, 2453–2467.

De Passillé, A.M., Christopherson, R. and Rushen, J. (1993) Nonnutritive sucking by the calf and postprandial secretion of insulin, CCK, and gastrin. *Physiology and Behavior* 54, 1069–1073.

De Passillé, A.M., Sweeney, B. and Rushen, J. (2010) Cross-sucking and gradual weaning of dairy calves. *Applied Animal Behaviour Science* 124, 11–15.

de Paula Vieira, A., Guesdon, V., de Passillé, A.M., von Keyserlingk, M.A.G. and Weary, D.M. (2008) Behavioural indicators of hunger in dairy calves. *Applied Animal Behaviour Science* 109, 180–189.

de Paula Vieira, A., von Keyserlingk, M.A.G. and Weary, D.M. (2010) Effects of pair versus single housing on performance and behavior of dairy calves before and after weaning from milk. *Journal of Dairy Science* 93, 3079–3085.

EFSA (2006) Scientific Opinion on the risks of poor welfare in intensive calf farming systems. An update of the Scientific Veterinary Committee Report on the Welfare of Calves. *The EFSA Journal* 366, 1–36.

Gaillard, C., Meagher, R.K., von Keyserlingk, M.A.G. and Weary, D.M. (2014) Social housing improves dairy calves' performance in two cognitive tests. *PLoS ONE* 9, e90205.

Gottardo, F., Mattiello, S., Cozzi, G., Canali, E., Scanziani, E., Ravarotto, L., Ferrante, V., Verga, M. and Andrighetto, I. (2002) The provision of drinking water to veal calves for welfare purposes. *Journal of Animal Science* 80, 2362–2372.

Hickey, M.C., Drennan, M. and Earley, B. (2003) The effect of abrupt weaning of suckler calves on the plasma concentrations of cortisol, catecholamines, leukocytes, acute-phase proteins and in vitro interferon-gamma production. *Journal of Animal Science* 81, 2847–2855.

Jasper, J., Budzynska, M. and Weary, D.M. (2008) Weaning distress in dairy calves: acute behavioural responses by limit-fed calves. *Applied Animal Behaviour Science* 110, 136–143.

Johnson, K., Burn, C.C. and Wathes, D.C. (2011) Rates and risk factors for contagious disease and mortality in young dairy heifers. *CAB Reviews: Perspectives in Agriculture, Veterinary Science, Nutrition and Natural Resources* 6, 59.

Jung, J. and Lidfors, L. (2001) Effects of amount of milk, milk flow and access to a rubber teat on cross-sucking and non-nutritive sucking in dairy calves. *Applied Animal Behaviour Science* 72, 201–213.

Kertz, A.F., Reutzel, L.F. and Mahoney, J.H. (1984) Ad libitum water intake by neonatal calves and its relationship to starter intake, weight gain, feces score and season. *Journal of Dairy Science* 67, 2964–2969.

Khan, M.A., Bach, A., Weary, D.M. and von Keyserlingk, M.A.G. (2016) Invited review: Transitioning from milk to solid feed in dairy heifers. *Journal of Dairy Science* 99, 885–902.

Lago, A., McGuirk, S.M., Bennett, T.B., Cook, N.B. and Nordlund, K.V. (2006) Calf respiratory disease and pen microenvironments in naturally ventilated calf barns in winter. *Journal of Dairy Science* 89, 4014–4025.

Losinger, W.C. and Heinrichs, A.J. (1997) Management practices associated with high mortality among preweaned dairy heifers. *Journal of Dairy Research* 64, 1–11.

McGuirk, S.M. (2011) Management of dairy calves from birth to weaning. In: Risco, C.A. and Melendez Retamal, P. (eds) *Dairy Production Medicine*. Wiley-Blackwell, Ames, IA, USA, pp. 175–193.

Moore, M., Tyler, J.W., Chigerwe, M., Dawes, M.E. and Middleton, J.R. (2005) Effect of delayed colostrum collection on colostral IgG concentration in dairy cows. *Journal of the American Veterinary Medical Association* 226, 1375–1377.

Olson, D.P., Papsian, C.J. and Ritter, R.C. (1980) The effects of cold stress on neonatal calves II. Absorption of colostral immunoglobulins. *Canadian Journal of Comparative Medicine* 44, 19–23.

Roland, L., Drillich, M., Klein-Jöbstl, D. and Iwersen, M. (2016) Invited review: Influence of climatic conditions on the development, performance, and health of calves. *Journal of Dairy Science* 99, 2438–2452.

Roth, B.A., Keil, N.M., Gygax, L. and Hillmann, E. (2009) Temporal distribution of sucking behavior in diary calves and influence of energy balance. *Applied Animal Behaviour Science* 119, 137–142.

Soberon, F., Raffrenato, E., Everett, R.W. and Van Amburgh, M.E. (2012) Preweaning milk replacer intake and effects on long-term productivity of dairy calves. *Journal of Dairy Science* 95, 783–793.

Teagasc (2017) Development of the calf digestive system. In: *Teagasc Calf Rearing Manual.* Agriculture and Food Development Authority, Teagasc, Carlow, Ireland, pp. 59–76.

Teagasc (2017) Calf diagnosis and disease prevention. In: *Teagasc Calf Rearing Manual.* Agriculture and Food Development Authority, Teagasc, Carlow, Ireland, pp. 97–122.

Wenge, J., Steinhöfel, I., Heinrich, C., Coenen, M. and Bachmann, L (2014) Water and concentrate intake, weight gain and duration of diarrhea in young suckling calves on different diets. *Livestock Science* 159, 133–140.

Index

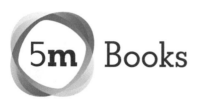
5m Books

Our new company 5m Books Ltd was formed in August 2020 and includes the books of 5m Publishing and Nottingham University Press.

Our mission is to publish the highest quality books in veterinary and animal sciences, agriculture, and aquaculture.

Join us at www.5mbooks.com or follow us on Twitter at @5m_Books to be part of our community and to find out more about our books and authors.

**If you an idea for a new book in a subject area in which we publish, we would be delighted to hear from you, please email us:
hello@5mbooks.com**

www.5mbooks.com

@5mBooks | @5m_Books | @5m_Books
linkedin.com/company/5mbooks